WF140S9A

OXFORD MEDI

D0524996

Respiratory Disease

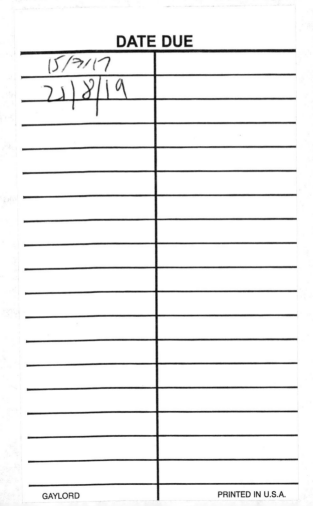

DATE DUE

15/7/17	
21/8/19	

Oxford Specialist Handbooks published and forthcoming

General Oxford Specialist Handbooks
A Resuscitation Room Guide
Addiction Medicine
Perioperative Medicine,
Second Edition
Post-Operative Complications,
Second edition

Oxford Specialist Handbooks in Anaesthesia
Cardiac Anaesthesia
General Thoracic Anaesthesia
Neuroanaesthesia
Obstetric Anaesthesia
Paediatric Anaesthesia
Regional Anaesthesia,
Stimulation and Ultrasound
Techniques

Oxford Specialist Handbooks in Cardiology
Adult Congenital Heart
Disease
Cardiac Catheterization and
Coronary Intervention
Echocardiography
Fetal Cardiology
Heart Failure
Hypertension
Nuclear Cardiology
Pacemakers and ICDs

Oxford Specialist Handbooks in Critical Care
Advanced Respiratory
Critical Care

Oxford Specialist Handbooks in End of Life Care
End of Life Care in Cardiology
End of Life Care in Dementia
End of Life Care in Nephrology
End of Life Care in Respiratory
Disease
End of Life Care in the Intensive
Care Unit

Oxford Specialist Handbooks in Neurology
Epilepsy
Parkinson's Disease and Other
Movement Disorders
Stroke Medicine

Oxford Specialist Handbooks in Paediatrics
Paediatric Endocrinology and
Diabetes
Paediatric Dermatology
Paediatric Gastroenterology,
Hepatology, and Nutrition
Paediatric Haematology and
Oncology
Paediatric Nephrology
Paediatric Neurology
Paediatric Radiology
Paediatric Respiratory Medicine

Oxford Specialist Handbooks in Psychiatry
Child and Adolescent Psychiatry
Old Age Psychiatry

Oxford Specialist Handbooks in Radiology
Interventional Radiology
Musculoskeletal Imaging

Oxford Specialist Handbooks in Surgery
Cardiothoracic Surgery
Hand Surgery
Hepato-pancreatobiliary Surgery
Oral Maxillo Facial Surgery
Neurosurgery
Operative Surgery, Second Edition
Otolaryngology and Head and
Neck Surgery
Plastic and Reconstructive Surgery
Surgical Oncology
Urological Surgery
Vascular Surgery

Respiratory Disease

From advanced disease to bereavement

Anna Spathis

Macmillian Consultant in Palliative Medicine
Cambridge University Hospitals NHS Foundation Trust,
Cambridge, UK

Helen E. Davies

Consultant in Respiratory Medicine
University Hospital Llandough
Cardiff and Vale University Health Board
Penarth, Cardiff, UK

Sara Booth

Clinical Director and Macmillan Consultant
in Palliative Medicine
Associate Lecturer, University of Cambridge, and
Honorary Senior Lecturer, Department of Palliative
Care and Policy, King's College, London, UK

Series Editor

Max Watson

Consultant in Palliative Medicine
Northern Ireland Hospice
Belfast, UK, and
Honorary Consultant
The Princess Alice Hospice
Esher, UK

OXFORD
UNIVERSITY PRESS

OXFORD
UNIVERSITY PRESS

Great Clarendon Street, Oxford OX2 6DP

Oxford University Press is a department of the University of Oxford.
It furthers the University's objective of excellence in research, scholarship,
and education by publishing worldwide in

Oxford New York

Auckland Cape Town Dar es Salaam Hong Kong Karachi
Kuala Lumpur Madrid Melbourne Mexico City Nairobi
New Delhi Shanghai Taipei Toronto

With offices in

Argentina Austria Brazil Chile Czech Republic France Greece
Guatemala Hungary Italy Japan Poland Portugal Singapore
South Korea Switzerland Thailand Turkey Ukraine Vietnam

Oxford is a registered trade mark of Oxford University Press
in the UK and in certain other countries

Published in the United States
by Oxford University Press Inc., New York

British Library Cataloguing in Publication Data
Data available

Library of Congress Cataloging in Publication Data
Data available

Typeset by Glyph International, Bangalore, India
Printed in Great Britain
on acid-free paper by
Ashford Colour Press Ltd, Gosport, Hampshire

ISBN 978–0–19–956403–3

10 9 8 7 6 5 4 3 2 1

Preface

It is a duty and a privilege to be able to provide compassionate and effective care from diagnosis to death.

Provision of end of life care for those with advanced respiratory disease is challenging, both in terms of the number of patients and the extent of their suffering. Lung cancer is the commonest malignant cause of death and COPD the fifth commonest cause of death worldwide. Quality of life is particularly poor, those with chronic, non-malignant respiratory disease appearing to suffer as much, if not more, than those with lung cancer. Uncontrolled symptoms tend to persist through a long and unpredictable functional decline, often compounded by psychological morbidity and social isolation.

Despite the magnitude of the problem, end of life care in respiratory disease has, until recently, been relatively neglected. Only in the last decade has there been gathering international acknowledgement that end of life care is an integral part of respiratory medicine. Respiratory specialists, in collaboration with palliative care colleagues, have a central role in ensuring that the care of those with advanced respiratory disease improves to the level of the best.

This concise and practical handbook aims both to guide respiratory specialists through the process of providing highest quality of end of life care, and to familiarise palliative care specialists with the unique problems faced by those with respiratory disease. We have attempted to improve our own clinical practice in respiratory and palliative medicine, by reviewing the evidence underpinning this field. We share with you the synthesis of this evidence-base, combined with our own clinical experience of caring for patients with end-stage respiratory disease. We hope this book will relieve the sense of helplessness often felt by professionals caring for patients in the last months, weeks and days of life.

We have learned much from our patients and their families, and we hope that this book, in turn, can contribute in its own small way to improving the care that those with advanced respiratory disease receive in the future.

Contents

Contents

Symbols and abbreviations

~	approximately
≡	equivalent to
↑	increased
±	plus/minus
📖	refer to
α	alpha
β	beta
Δ	delta
δ	delta
κ	kappa
μ	mu
5HT	5-hydroxytryptamine (receptors)
A-a	alveolar to arterial
ABG	arterial blood gas
ACE	angiotensin-converting enzyme
ACP	advance care planning
ACTH	adrenocorticotropic hormone
ADA	After Death Analysis
ADRT	advance decision to refuse treatment
ADH	antidiuretic hormone
ADL	activity of daily living
AHP	allied health professionals
AIP	acute interstitial pneumonia
ALS	amyotrophic lateral sclerosis
AMP	adenosine monophosphate
ATP	adenosine triphosphate
AV	atrioventricular
BAC	bronchoalveolar cell
BBB	blood-brain barrier
bd	twice daily
BDZ	benzodiazepines
BE	base excess
BMI	body mass index
BSC	best supportive care
BTS	British Thoracic Society
CAV	cyclophosphamide, doxorubicin, and vincristine

CBT	cognitive behavioural therapy
CF	cystic fibrosis
CFA	cryptogenic fibrosing alveolitis
CFTR	cystic fibrosis transmembrane conductance regulator
CHART	continuous hyperfractionated accelerated radiotherapy
COP	cryptogenic organizing pneumonia
COPD	chronic obstructive pulmonary disease
CPR	cardiopulmonary resuscitation
CRD	chronic respiratory disease
CRP	C-reactive protein
CSCI	continuous subcutaneous infusion
CT	computerized (axial) tomography
CTEPH	chronic thromboembolic pulmonary hypertension
CTPA	computerized tomographic pulmonary angiogram
CVA	cerebrovascular accident
CXR	chest X-ray
DIP	desquamative interstitial pneumonia
DNAR	do not attempt resuscitation (decision)
DPLD	diffuse parenchymal lung disease
DSM-IV	*Diagnostic and Statistical Manual of Mental Disorders, 4th edition*
DVT	deep vein thrombosis
ECG	electrocardiography/electrocardiogram
EGFR	epidermal growth factor receptor
EMG	electromyography
EOLC	end of life care
EPP	extrapleural pneumonectomy
ET	endotracheal
F	French (unit of measurement)
FBC	full blood count
FEV1	forced expiratory volume in 1 second
FFM	fat-free mass
FNA	fine needle aspiration
FPAH	familial pulmonary arterial hypertension
FVC	forced vital capacity
GFR	glomerular filtration rate
GI	gastrointestinal
GMC	General Medical Council
GORD	gastro-oesophageal reflux disease
GP	general practitioner

GSF	Gold Standards Framework
HDU	high dependency unit
HIV	human immunodeficiency virus
HP	hypersensitivity pneumonitis
HRCT	high resolution CT
IASLC	International Association for the Study of Lung Cancer
ICP	intracranial pressure
ICSD	International Classification of Sleep Disorders
IIDB	Industrial Injuries Disablement Benefit
IIP	idiopathic interstitial pneumonia
IL1	interleukin-1
IL6	interleukin-6
IL8	interleukin-8
ILD	interstitial lung disease
IM	intramuscular
INR	international normalized ratio
IPAH	idiopathic pulmonary arterial hypertension
IPF	idiopathic pulmonary fibrosis
IR	immediate release
IRT	immunoreactive trypsin
IT	information technology
ITU	intensive therapy unit
IV	intravenous
JVP	jugular venous pressure
kg	kilogram
LAM	lymphangioleiomyomatosis
LC	lung cancer
LCH	Langerhans cell histiocytosis
LCP	Liverpool Care Pathway for the Dying Patient
LDH	lactate dehydrogenase
LEMS	Lambert-Eaton myasthenic syndrome
LIP	lymphoid interstitial pneumonia
LMWH	low molecular weight heparin
LPA	lasting power of attorney
LTOT	long-term oxygen therapy
LVRS	lung volume reduction surgery
M3G	morphine-3-glucuronide
M6G	morphine-6-glucuronide
MCA	Mental Capacity Act
mcg	microgram

MDT	multidisciplinary team
mg	milligram
MI	myocardial infarction
mL	milliliter
MND	motor neurone disease
MPE	malignant pleural effusion
MR	modified release
MRC	Medical Research Council
MRI	magnetic resonance imaging
N+V	nausea and vomiting
NA	noradrenaline
NAC	N-acetylcysteine
NaSSA	noradrenergic and specific serotonergic antidepressant
NCPC	National Council for Palliative Care
NHL	non-Hodgkin's lymphoma
NICE	National Institute for Health and Clinical Excellence
NIPPV	non-invasive positive pressure ventilation/ventilator
NIV	non-invasive ventilation
NMDA	N-methyl-D-aspartic acid (receptor)
NMES	neuromuscular electrical stimulation
nocte	at night
NRS	numerical rating scale
NRT	nicotine replacement therapy
NT-proBNP	N-terminal prohormone brain natriuretic peptide
NSAID	non-steroidal anti-inflammatory drug
NSCLC	non-small cell lung cancer
NSIP	nonspecific interstitial pneumonia
NYHA	New York Heart Association
od	once daily
OSA	obstructive sleep apnoea
OT	occupational therapist
PA	posteroanterior
$PaCO_2$	arterial partial pressure of carbon dioxide
PaO_2	arterial partial pressure of oxygen
PAP	pulmonary arterial pressure
PCP	pneumocystis carinii (now jiroveci) pneumonia
PDE	phosphodiesterase
PE	pulmonary embolism
PET	positron emission tomography
PH	pulmonary hypertension

po	oral
PPC	preferred priorities of care
PPH	primary pulmonary hypertension
PPS	post-polio syndrome
prn	as needed
PTH	parathyroid hormone
PTHrP	parathyroid hormone-related peptide
PTSD	post-traumatic stress disorder
qds	four times a day
RB-ILD	respiratory bronchiolitis associated interstitial lung disease
RCT	randomized controlled trial
REM	rapid eye movement
RR	relative risk
SBOT	short-burst oxygen therapy
sc	subcutaneous
SCLC	small cell lung cancer
SCR	Supportive Care Register
SD	syringe driver
SIADH	syndrome of inappropriate ADH secretion
SL	sublingual
SSRI	selective serotonin reuptake inhibitor
SVC	superior vena cava
SVCO	superior vena cava obstruction
TB	tuberculosis
TCA	tricyclic antidepressant
tds	three times daily
TD	transdermal
TENS	transcutaneous electrical nerve stimulation
TGF-α	transforming growth factor-alpha
TLCO	carbon monoxide transfer factor
TM	transmucosal
TNF-α	tumour necrosis factor-α
TNF-β	tumour necrosis factor-β
TNM	Tumour/Node/Metastasis (system)
UIP	usual interstitial pneumonia
USS	ultrasound scan
UTI	urinary tract infection
VATS	video-assisted thoracoscopic surgery
VC	vital capacity
V/Q	ventilation/perfusion

VTE	venous thromboembolism
WFI	water for injection
WHO	World Health Organization

Chapter 1

End-stage respiratory disease

The burden of end-stage respiratory disease

Respiratory disease is a major public health problem. Advances in available treatments have prolonged the life expectancy for many chronic lung conditions. As survival increases, so does the burden of patient morbidity and the adverse impact on patients' quality of life. In turn, the demand on healthcare services is intensifying.

The morbidity from non-malignant respiratory conditions is at least as severe, if not more so, than that from advanced malignant disease. Non-malignant diseases impose a heavy symptom burden, reduce quality of life significantly, and may have a worse prognosis from time of diagnosis than many solid tumours. In addition, many such diseases, such as cystic fibrosis (CF), interstitial lung disease (ILD), and pulmonary hypertension (PH), occur in young people with dependants. The difficulties and strains imposed on carers of those with advanced respiratory disease are frequently overlooked, and referral to specialist palliative care is rare despite the level of physical symptoms and psychosocial need.

A significant proportion of the treatment options for chronic respiratory disease are not disease-modifying. Management decisions are often complex, and where a radical treatment (such as lung transplantation) is available, it is usually only suitable for highly selected patients, such as those who are still relatively fit and near the time of diagnosis.

Many respiratory teams now try to provide supportive care with a multi-professional approach from the time of diagnosis, to help reduce or contain the psychosocial as well as the physical impact of the disease. This is critically important in conditions such as CF or chronic obstructive pulmonary disease (COPD), where the patient and their family may live with the consequences of the illness for many years.

Prevalence

- Respiratory disease is the second most prevalent cause of death worldwide.
- In the UK, respiratory disease accounts for one in five deaths.
- COPD is predicted to be the third leading cause of death globally by 2020.
- Lung cancer is the most common cancer in the world, and claims almost a quarter of all cancer-related deaths in the UK.
- There is a significant variation in respiratory disease mortality between different social classes:
  - 44% of respiratory deaths are associated with social class inequality.
  - Mortality is greater for men in unskilled manual occupations than those in professional roles, particularly in those with COPD and tuberculosis (TB).
- Over the next decade, chronic respiratory disease is predicted to increase by 30% in developing countries if preventative strategies, such as smoking prevention, are not employed.

Table 1.1 Leading causes of death in UK and USA (World Health Organisation, WHO 2004)
http:// www.who.int/mediacentre/factsheets/fs310/en/index.html

Cause of death	Percentage
Coronary heart disease	16.3
Stroke and other cerebrovascular diseases	9.3
Trachea/bronchus/lung Cancers	5.9
Lower respiratory infections	3.8
Chronic Obstructive Pulmonary Disease (COPD)	3.5
Alzheimer's and other dementias	3.4

Disease trajectories

The key challenge in providing end of life care to patients with advanced non-malignant disease, such as chronic obstructive pulmonary disease, is the difficulty in prognosticating caused by the unpredictable disease trajectory.

Significant variation exists between the expected disease trajectories of different respiratory illnesses, and between the trajectory of cancer and non-cancer causes of death.

Classification

Three main illness trajectories have been described:
- Initial preservation of function with subsequent short period of decline in the advanced stages e.g. cancer (Figure 1.1a).
  - The timing of death can often be anticipated and appropriate preparations made.
- Long-term limitation ('organ failure') with intermittent acute episodes or 'entry-reentry' pattern e.g. COPD, pulmonary fibrosis (Figure 1.1b).
  - An inexorable decline in function and health-related quality of life is typically seen, punctuated by intermittent exacerbations that may be associated with hospitalization.
  - In comparison to patients with malignant disease, the functional level at diagnosis tends to be lower and the overall trajectory longer in duration.
  - The trajectory can be highly variable, and the timing of the terminal event particularly unpredictable.
  - Prognostication for patients with this illness trajectory is difficult and makes provision of good end of life care (EOLC) challenging. It is often not clear when advance care planning should start and, if the proximity to end of life is misjudged, there may not be time to initiate adequate input/support or determine the patient's wishes and preferences for care (see 📖 Chapter 4 pp. 52–54).
- Gradual deterioration on background of prior poor functioning e.g. frailty, dementia (Figure 1.1c).

Distinguishing between distinct trajectories can help to shape the provision of physical, psychosocial, and spiritual care for individual patients tailored towards their expected end of life needs.

It must be remembered that not all patients will adhere to a predicted disease course, and many patients will have dual pathology e.g. lung cancer and COPD.

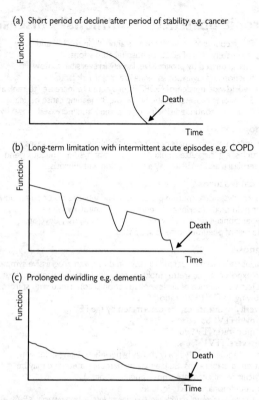

Fig. 1.1 Typical disease trajectories for progressive chronic illness. (adapted from Murray *et al*[1]. with permission from BMJ Publishing Group Ltd.)

Reference

1. Murray SA, Kendall M, Boyd K, Sheikh A (2005) Clinical review: Illness trajectories and palliative care. *BMJ*; 330: 1007–1011.

Chronic obstructive pulmonary disease

- COPD accounts for >30,000 deaths annually in the UK and approximately 10% of all acute hospital admissions.
- It is characterized by progressive, largely irreversible airflow obstruction and cigarette smoking is a major risk factor.
- The worldwide burden of COPD is projected to increase (to rank as the 5th leading cause of disability and the 3rd leading cause of death by 2020) due to continued risk factor exposure and increased longevity.

Pathogenesis

- An abnormal inflammatory response to inhaled noxious gases or particles, e.g. cigarette smoke, results in emphysema, mucous gland hyperplasia, and small airway inflammation with fibrosis.

Clinical features

- Cough, dyspnoea, sputum production, and wheeze occur commonly.
- Cor pulmonale (peripheral oedema) or respiratory failure (hypercapnia-induced early morning headaches) may develop.
- The risk of pneumothorax is increased.

Diagnosis

- Diagnosis is often suspected clinically in those with progressive symptoms and exposure to cigarette smoke or environmental/occupational dusts.
- Objective evidence of airflow obstruction is confirmed with spirometry showing an FEV1/FVC ratio <0.7.
- Severity of disease can be determined by the FEV1:
  - mild: FEV1 50–80%
  - moderate: FEV1 30–50%
  - severe: FEV1 <30%.
- Chest radiography typically shows hyperinflated lung fields with flattened diaphragms. Bullae may be demonstrated (and may be difficult to differentiate from a pneumothorax).
- Extra-pulmonary effects include:
  - *Cachexia, skeletal-muscle wasting, weight loss:* A body weight <90% predicted is a marker for increased mortality. Both systemic inflammation and oxidative stress are thought to play a role in loss of fat-free mass (FFM) and muscle wasting. Pro-inflammatory cytokines (i.e. tumour necrosis factor-α (TNF-α), interleukin-6 (IL6), and interleukin-8 (IL8)) are increased in COPD patients with weight loss compared to those of similar disease severity without weight loss. Poor dietary intake and repeated infections also contribute.
  - *Increased incidence of cardiovascular disease:* The exact mechanism has not yet been elucidated. However, smoking, hypoxaemia, systemic inflammation e.g. raised C-reactive protein (CRP), and cardio-stimulatory medication e.g. β-agonists or anticholinergics are thought to play a role.
  - *Osteoporosis:* The aetiology of bone loss is diverse but includes use of corticosteroids, systemic inflammation and oxidative stress, malnutrition and low body mass index (BMI), smoking, and a sedentary lifestyle.

- *Mood and sleep disorders:* Over 50% of patients report depressive symptoms at some point in their disease. Anxiety and insomnia are common and contribute to chronic fatigue, which exacerbates patients' impaired functional status.

Treatment

General

- Smoking cessation:
  - This is the most effective tool in reducing decline in FEV1 and sputum production, and preserving level of physical function.
  - Smoking cessation returns rate of FEV1 decline to that of a non-smoker.
  - Use the 'Five As' approach, in tandem with patient support from the primary care team:
    - ask if smoking at every visit
    - advise to quit at every visit
    - assess readiness to quit
    - assist in smoking cessation
    - arrange for follow-up.
  - Nicotine replacement therapy (NRT) minimizes withdrawal symptoms. Patches, lozenges, chewing gum, tablets, nasal sprays, and inhaler preparations are all available. Non-NRT e.g. bupropion reduces nicotine cravings through its effect on dopamine, serotonin, and noradrenaline neurotransmission. Both NRT and non-NRT are best used as an adjunct to motivational support.
- Optimize body weight.
- Encourage regular exercise:
  - Reduction in physical activity is associated with a poorer prognosis and increased risk of hospital admission.
- Influenza and pneumococcal vaccination.
- Consider osteoporosis prophylaxis:
  - Calcium and vitamin D.
  - Bisphosphonate therapy.

Medical

Pharmacological treatment in patients with COPD aims to reduce symptoms and exacerbation frequency, rather than modify the underlying disease. A suggested step-wise approach is outlined below.

- Bronchodilators:
  - Initially a short-acting β2 agonist should be used e.g. inhaled salbutamol via a spacer device.
  - If still symptomatic, add a short-acting anticholinergic e.g. ipratropium.
  - Persistent symptoms may require a regular long-acting bronchodilator, either an anticholinergic (e.g. tiotropium) or a β2 agonist (e.g. salmeterol). Short-acting anticholinergics should be stopped prior to initiation of long-acting anticholinergic agents.
  - Addition of oral methylxanthines (e.g. theophylline) may improve symptoms, but their use needs to be weighed against the risk of adverse effects (e.g. nausea, tachyarrhythmia).

- Corticosteroids:
  - Consider a trial of inhaled corticosteroid in patients with an FEV1 ≤50% and ≥2 exacerbations per year e.g. beclometasone 400mcg bd. This may reduce exacerbation frequency but has no impact on lung function decline. Discontinue if no clinical benefit after 4 weeks.
  - Oral steroids should not be routinely prescribed in stable patients with severe disease. However, if unable to withdraw following exacerbation, use the lowest dose tolerated.
- Mucolytic agents:
  - Mucolytic agents (e.g. carbocisteine 750mg tds) can improve symptoms in patients with viscous sputum.
- Oxygen therapy:
  - Ambulatory oxygen via a cylinder may be useful in mobile patients on long-term oxygen therapy (LTOT) or in those with symptomatic exertional oxygen desaturation.
  - LTOT via a concentrator is given after formal assessment, to improve survival in patients with respiratory failure. It is indicated in patients with a PaO_2 of <7.3kPa (55mmHg) when stable, or <8.0kPa in the presence of peripheral oedema, secondary polycythaemia, nocturnal hypoxaemia, or pulmonary hypertension. Oxygen should be used for >15hrs/d (including sleep).
- Symptom palliation (see 📖 Chapter 5 for details):
  - Breathlessness can be palliated with non-drug measures, such as breathing and relaxation techniques, energy conservation, and use of a fan, as well as with pharmacological approaches, such as use of opioids.
  - Treatment of other prevalent symptoms, such as anxiety and depression, is vital.

Pulmonary rehabilitation
- This provides a multidisciplinary programme of physical conditioning, breathing retraining, education, and psychological support.
- It has been shown to improve exercise capacity, subjective dyspnoea, and quality of life; reduce hospitalizations and healthcare utilization; and decrease anxiety and depression (see 📖 Chapter 5 p. 68 for further details).

Surgical
- Bullectomy reduces dyspnoea and improves lung function if a large bulla is present (>1/3 hemithorax).
- Lung volume reduction surgery (LVRS) may be of use in highly selected patients. The greatest benefit is seen in those with upper lobe emphysema and low exercise capacity.

Lung transplantation
- COPD is the most common indication for transplantation.
- Consider in selected patients <60y for bilateral lung and <65y for single lung transplant if FEV1 <20% predicted, hypercapnic (≥6.5mmHg), resting hypoxaemia (<6.0mmHg), rapid clinical decline (i.e. frequent exacerbations and poor quality of life), or pulmonary hypertension. Transplantation rates are limited by donor shortage.

Future approaches
- One-way endobronchial valves offer a potential alternative to LVRS. They are inserted bronchoscopically into areas of severe emphysema and prevent air entering these segments but allow its release and escape of secretions. Ventilation-perfusion matching is improved, as air is redirected to less diseased areas of lung.

Lung cancer

- Lung cancer is the most common cause of cancer mortality worldwide for both men and women.
- In the UK >36,000 cases are diagnosed annually and one person dies of lung cancer every 15 minutes.
- The male: female sex ratio is 2:1.
- In the UK and US, male lung cancer mortality rates are declining and female rates have reached a plateau. However, in developing countries levels are increasing due to endemic tobacco use.

Risk factors

- Cigarette smoking:
  - Smoking accounts for approximately 90% of lung cancer cases.
  - The lung cancer risk is proportional to lifetime cigarette consumption. A 75-year-old male lifelong smoker has a cumulative risk of 16% for developing lung cancer. However, if he ceased smoking at age 60, 50, 40, or 30y this risk would reduce to 10%, 6%, 3% or 2% respectively. The overall relative risk for lung cancer in a current smoker is 10–30 times that of someone who has never smoked.
  - Cigar (relative risk (RR) ~2–5 times that of someone who has never smoked) and pipe smoking (RR ~5 times) both increase risk, but less than cigarettes. Passive smoking increases risk in non-smokers.
- Occupational and environmental exposures e.g. asbestos, radon, wood smoke:
  - The risk of lung cancer in smokers with asbestos exposure is multiplicative (RR ~55–60 times); presence of asbestosis is also associated with an increased lung cancer rate.
- Pulmonary fibrosis:
  - This is associated with an increased relative risk of lung cancer of approximately 8–14 times.

Types of lung cancer

Non-small cell lung cancer (NSCLC) (75–80%)

Subtypes include:

- Adenocarcinoma (~35%):
  - This is the most common tumour type in both smokers and never-smokers; it is often peripherally situated.
  - Bronchoalveolar cell (BAC) carcinoma is a histologically distinct subtype of adenocarcinoma that may present with profuse sputum production (bronchorrhoea).
- Squamous cell carcinoma (~30%):
  - Incidence positively correlates with smoking history; typically originates in central airways and may cavitate.
- Large cell carcinoma (~10%).
- Adenosquamous.

Small cell lung cancer (SCLC) (20–25%)

- SCLC is often disseminated at the time of presentation.

Others (5%)
- Bronchopulmonary neuroendocrine (carcinoid) tumours (2.5%):
  - Most are 'typical' with low metastatic potential; ~10% are 'atypical' with more aggressive histological and clinical features.
- Pulmonary lymphoma, sarcomas, and adenoid cystic carcinomas are rare.

Clinical features
- Many patients have non-specific features and may be found to have lung cancer incidentally on imaging performed for another indication.
- Symptoms may be due to the local tumour itself, metastatic disease, or paraneoplastic phenomena (Table 1.2).

Table 1.2 Symptoms and signs of lung cancer

Local effects	Distant effects	Paraneoplastic syndromes
Cough	Anorexia, weight loss, cachexia	Clubbing
Dyspnoea	Cervical/supraclavicular lymphadenopathy	Hypercalcaemia (see Chapter 6)
Haemoptysis	Bone pain/pathological fractures	Syndrome of Inappropriate ADH (SIADH)*
Chest pain	Hypercoagulability	Ectopic ACTH (Cushing's syndrome)*
Recurrent/unresolving pneumonia	Fatigue	Lambert-Eaton myasthenic syndrome*
Wheeze/stridor	Headache, confusion	Hypertrophic pulmonary osteo-arthropathy
Pleural effusion		Dermatomyositis/ polymyositis
Hoarse voice		Cerebellar syndrome*
Dysphagia		Limbic encephalitis*
SVCO (see Chapter 6)		
Horner's syndrome		
Pancoast's syndrome		

*Occur mainly with SCLC

Investigations in advanced disease
CXR (PA and lateral)
- This may demonstrate disease progression, bony involvement, or pleural effusion.

Blood tests
- Biochemistry:
  - Hyponatraemia secondary to SIADH is most common in SCLC.
  - Hypercalcaemia is again more common in SCLC.
  - Hypokalaemic alkalosis and hyperglycaemia may arise due to ectopic ACTH production, particularly in SCLC or carcinoid tumours. Marked elevation of 24h urinary free-cortisol and plasma ACTH levels are seen.
  - Liver test abnormalities may be seen with hepatic involvement.

Imaging
- CT neck, chest, liver, and adrenals allows staging of the extent of disease.
- Isotope bone scanning and CT brain should be performed if metastases are clinically suspected.

Histocytological diagnosis
- Pleural fluid cytology:
  - The presence of malignant cells within pleural fluid renders the underlying lung tumour inoperable. However, an inflammatory effusion secondary to an obstructing lesion or complicating pneumonia does not. Differentiation is therefore important in guiding management, and pleural fluid analysis ± thoracoscopy should always be undertaken in patients who develop a pleural effusion but are otherwise potential candidates for tumour resection.

Staging

The stage of disease often determines the treatment offered to patients. NSCLC is characterized using the Tumour/Node/Metastasis (TNM) system graded I–IV (Table 1.3). Approximately 45% of patients have stage IV disease on presentation.

SCLC is classified as either limited (confined to ipsilateral hemithorax) or extensive.

Treatment

Management is governed by histological type and stage of disease, and patients' performance status and wishes.

The multidisciplinary team should always be involved, with a chest physician, lung nurse specialist, radiologist, thoracic surgeon, oncologist, palliative medicine specialist, and pathologist present, to discuss appropriate care for individual patients.

Best supportive care (BSC)
- Best supportive care is the unified approach to management of any disease, to enable patients to live optimally through all stages of their illness whilst maximizing treatment and minimizing suffering.
- It embraces pre-diagnosis, diagnosis, intended treatment phase (potential cure, disease regression, or relapse), continued illness or co-morbidity, death, and bereavement.
- Physical, psychological, social, spiritual, cultural, and financial support should be given to maximize quality of life of all patients regardless of underlying disease or stage.

NSCLC

Surgery

Surgery can offer a potential chance of cure. Tumour resectability and patients' fitness for surgery need to be considered prior to attempted excision. Current resection rates in the UK (11%) are lower than in the rest of Europe (17%) and North America (21%).

Chemotherapy

This improves quality of life and median survival (usually by 6–8 weeks) compared to best supportive care in patients of performance status 0–2. A two-drug platinum-based combination is recommended e.g. cisplatin and gemcitabine. There is no consensus on the use of adjuvant and neo-adjuvant chemotherapy. Novel targeted drugs such as epidermal growth factor receptor (EGFR) antagonists (e.g. Erlotinib) may be used in selected patients.

Radiotherapy

Radiotherapy can be given with curative intent, as continuous hyper-fractionated accelerated radiotherapy (CHART), or for local symptom control. It can control haemoptysis in up to 90% of cases, reduce dyspnoea and cough due to airway obstruction in approximately 60%, and minimize pain e.g. from bony metastases. Side effects include tiredness, oesophagitis at higher doses, skin soreness, loss of chest hair, and occasionally nausea and vomiting.

SCLC

- Combination chemotherapy: 80–90% response rate is seen in limited stage SCLC, and 60–80% if extensive disease. Treatment regimens include etoposide and cisplatin (or carboplatin), or cyclophosphamide, doxorubicin, and vincristine (CAV).
- Prophylactic cranial radiotherapy: can decrease risk of brain metastases and has been shown to improve 3y survival rates by 5.4% in limited stage disease. In extensive disease, it is recommended if there is a response to chemotherapy and a good performance status is maintained.

Prognosis

This is related to the stage of disease at presentation.

NSCLC

- The median survival for patients with metastatic disease is 6 months.
- In early stage IA disease, 5y survival rates are ~73%.
- In stage II, III, and IV disease, 5y survival rates are 22–34%, 3–13%, and 1–2% respectively.

SCLC

- Limited stage disease: median survival 15–20 months; 5y survival 10–13%.
- Extensive stage disease: median survival 8–13 months; 5y survival 1–2%.

Table 1.3 TNM classification for Lung Cancer Staging, 7th edition (International Association for the Study of Lung Cancer (IASLC))

Primary tumour (T)

TX	Primary tumour cannot be assessed; or tumour proven by presence of malignant cells in sputum or bronchial washings but not visualised by imaging or bronchoscopy
T0	No evidence of primary tumour
TIS	Carcinoma *in situ*
T1	Tumour ≤ 3cm in its greatest dimension, surrounded by lung or visceral pleura, without bronchoscopic evidence of invasion more proximal than the lobar bronchus (i.e. not in the main bronchus)
T1a	Tumour ≤ 2cm in greatest dimension
T1b	Tumour > 2cm but ≤ 3cm in greatest dimension
T2	Tumour >3cm but ≤ 7cm; or tumour which (i) involves the main bronchus, ≥ 2cm distal to the carina, (ii) invades visceral pleura or (iii) is associated with atelectasis or obstructive pneumonitis that extends to the hilar region but does not involve the whole lung
T2a	Tumour > 3cm but ≤ 5cm in greatest dimension
T2b	Tumour > 5cm but ≤ 7cm
T3	Tumour >7cm; or tumour which directly invades chest wall (including superior sulcus tumours), diaphragm, parietal pericardium, phrenic nerve, mediastinal pleura; or tumour in the main bronchus < 2cm distal to the carina but without involvement of the carina; or associated atelectasis or obstructive pneumonitis of the entire lung; or separate tumour nodule(s) in the same lobe as the primary tumour
T4	Tumour of any size that invades: mediastinum, heart, great vessels, trachea, recurrent laryngeal nerve, oesophagus, vertebral body, carina; or separate tumour nodule(s) in another ipsilateral lobe

Regional lymph nodes (N)

NX	Cannot be assessed
N0	No regional lymph node metastasis
N1	Metastasis in ipsilateral peri-bronchial and/or ipsilateral hilar node(s) and intra-pulmonary nodes, including involvement by direct tumour extension
N2	Metastasis in ipsilateral mediastinal and/or subcarinal lymph node(s)
N3	Metastasis in contralateral mediastinal, contralateral hilar, or any scalene or supraclavicular node(s)

Table 1.3 (*Contd.*)

Distant metastasis (M)	
MX	Cannot be assessed
M0	No distant metastasis
M1	Distant metastasis
M1a	Separate tumour nodule(s) in a contralateral lobe; tumour with pleural nodules, or malignant pleural (or pericardial) effusion
M1b	Distant metastasis

Mesothelioma

Malignant mesothelioma is a primary neoplasm commonly arising from mesothelial cells lining the pleural surface (>90%) or peritoneum (7%), and less frequently the pericardium or tunica vaginalis. There is no cure. The annual incidence is increasing in Europe and is expected to peak in the UK in 2015. It affects males more commonly than females (approximately 4:1), and two-thirds of patients are diagnosed between the ages of 40 and 70 years. The main cause of mesothelioma is asbestos contact and a mean latency period of >20 years is seen between exposure and disease onset.

Clinical features
- Insidious breathlessness.
- Chest pain.
- Constitutional symptoms e.g. weight loss, anorexia, sweating, fatigue.
- Pleural effusion (in over 95% during disease course).
- Chest wall invasion (e.g. at pleural puncture sites).

Investigations
- Pleural fluid analysis: cytological yield from pleural fluid is low (~20%).
- Pleural biopsy: histological diagnosis may be obtained from either thoracoscopic or imaging-guided pleural biopsy.

Imaging
- CXR often reveals a pleural effusion or pleural thickening.
- CT scanning may suggest malignant pleural thickening (but cannot differentiate mesothelioma from secondary pleural malignancies). It can also show evidence of local invasion (e.g. chest wall, mediastinal) and features of prior asbestos exposure (e.g. pleural plaques). Distant metastases often occur late and are rarely clinically evident.

Types
- Epithelioid (50–60%); associated with a better prognosis.
- Sarcomatoid (~10%).
- Mixed (biphasic).

Staging
There is no universally agreed staging system for mesothelioma.

Management
- *Pleural effusion control:* More than 93% recur following drainage and early pleurodesis is appropriate. Use of an indwelling pleural catheter may be useful if the lung fails to re-expand (see 📖 Chapter 7 p. 160).
- *Chemotherapy:* Anti-folate agents e.g. pemetrexed, in combination with cisplatin, provide a survival advantage of approximately 3 months, and improve symptoms and quality of life.
- *Radiotherapy:* Use of routine prophylactic pleural puncture site radiotherapy to reduce rate of tumour seeding in mesothelioma is debated. It should be offered to patients with large pleural puncture sites (e.g. ≥24F thoracostomy or post-thoracoscopy), and those with symptomatic chest wall deposits.

- *Surgery:* Radical surgery e.g. extrapleural pneumonectomy (EPP) has not been shown to improve survival and is associated with a high mortality and post-operative morbidity.
- *Psychological support:* Many patients with mesothelioma will have prior knowledge of workmates who have succumbed to asbestos-related illness and will have lived with anxiety of a similar fate for many years. At diagnosis many patients will experience fear, uncertainty, anger, guilt, and resentment towards previous employers, and contact with a counsellor to talk about such emotions can be beneficial. Use of an anxiolytic or anti-depressant medication may also help (see 📖 Chapter 6 pp. 116–121).
- *Pain control* (see 📖 Chapter 6 pp. 94–110).
- *Nausea and vomiting; constipation* (see 📖 Chapter 6 pp. 132–136).
- *Excessive sweating:* This is not uncommon in mesothelioma. It may arise as a consequence of the cancer itself, drugs (e.g. opioids, steroids), co-existing infection, or anxiety. It can be a significant problem.
  - Treat possible contributory factors e.g. infection.
  - Adapt environment e.g. cooler room temperature, lighter bed linen, cotton clothing.
  - Drugs: paracetamol 1g qds, dexamethasone 2–4mg daily, and cimetidine 800mg nocte/bd may help. Anticholinergic agents such as hyoscine butylbromide 20mg tds or a hyoscine hydrobromide patch can be tried. Thalidomide 100–200mg nocte (acting through an inhibitory effect on cytokine production) should be reserved for specialist use in severe refractory cases only.
- *Intractable cough:*
  - Palliative radiotherapy, chemotherapy, and drainage of pleural effusion may improve cancer-related cough.
  - Anti-tussive medication can inhibit peripheral cough receptors (simple linctus or nebulized local anaesthetic e.g. bupivacaine 0.25% qds) or can act centrally (e.g. opioids such as codeine linctus 10mL or 30mg qds, methadone linctus 2.5–5mL, or morphine sulphate solution 2.5–5mg 4 hourly).
  - Baclofen 10mg qds, inhaled sodium cromoglicate 10mg (2 puffs) qds, and paroxetine all have a recognized anti-tussive effect.
  - Alternative non-malignant causes of cough should be addressed:
    - smoking cessation and bronchodilators for airways disease
    - stop pro-tussive medication (i.e. ACE inhibitors)
    - antacid therapy for gastro-oesophageal reflux
    - nasal decongestant/corticosteroids for post-nasal drip
    - steroids for cough related to concomitant asthma, COPD, or pulmonary fibrosis.
- *Legal and welfare issues:* Application for compensation and benefit entitlements for asbestos-related disease can provoke additional anxiety. An experienced solicitor should be contacted early. Eligibility for common law (civil) compensation depends on demonstrating a clear history of occupational asbestos exposure. In the UK, state compensation claims are made via the social service system e.g. Industrial Injuries Disablement Benefit (IIDB).

Prognosis

- Prognosis is related to patients' performance status and histological subtype; a good performance status and epithelioid histology are associated with a better prognosis. Other weaker poor prognostic indicators include age (>75 years), male gender, anaemia, thrombocythaemia, leucocytosis, raised lactate dehydrogenase (LDH) levels, significant weight loss, and chest pain.
- Overall the median survival is 8–14 months, although survival rates of >5 years have been reported.

Interstitial lung disease

Interstitial lung disease (ILD), or diffuse parenchymal lung disease (DPLD), primarily affects the lung interstitium. It represents a combination of underlying inflammatory and fibrotic lung disease and may be classified as idiopathic or secondary. Diagnosis is often achieved following clinical assessment and high resolution CT (HRCT) scanning, which may preclude the need for lung biopsy.

- Idiopathic interstitial pneumonia (IIP)—there are seven subtypes, each distinguished by clinical, radiological, and histopathological features:
  - usual interstitial pneumonia (UIP) or idiopathic pulmonary fibrosis (IPF)—previously known as cryptogenic fibrosing alveolitis (CFA)
  - nonspecific interstitial pneumonia (NSIP)
  - cryptogenic organizing pneumonia (COP)
  - desquamative interstitial pneumonia (DIP)
  - respiratory bronchiolitis associated interstitial lung disease (RB-ILD)
  - lymphoid interstitial pneumonia (LIP)
  - acute interstitial pneumonia (AIP).
- Secondary to underlying pathology including:
  - connective tissue disease including sarcoidosis
  - Langerhans cell histiocytosis (LCH)
  - lymphangioleiomyomatosis (LAM)
  - hypersensitivity pneumonitis (HP)
  - drug-induced pulmonary toxicity e.g. nitrofurantoin, amiodarone
  - infection
  - malignancy i.e. lymphoma, lymphangitis carcinomatosis
  - environmental/occupational exposures e.g. asbestosis.

Clinical features

- Progressive exertional dyspnoea and/or non-productive cough.
- Fine bibasal late inspiratory crackles on auscultation.
- Clubbing in up to 50% of patients.
- Cyanosis in advanced disease.

Management

- Good RCT data to guide treatment of the different subtypes of IIP are lacking. Recommended therapeutic approaches, focused on anti-inflammatory, immunosuppressive, and anti-oxidant agents, are summarized below.
- In all cases, concomitant infection, airways disease, and gastro-oesophageal reflux should be addressed. Opioids and benzodiazepines may aid relief of dyspnoea and cough (see 📖 Chapter 5 pp. 78–83).

UIP/IPF

Pharmacological management
- Prednisolone (tapering from 0.5mg/kg/day to 10–20mg/day) with azathioprine (2mg/kg, maximum 150mg/day) and N-acetylcysteine (NAC, 600mg tds) has been shown to have a significantly better treatment effect than prednisolone and azathioprine alone. An observed trial of treatment should be given, with early withdrawal of this regimen if deterioration is evident.

- Oxygen therapy can palliate breathlessness in some patients. An individual clinical assessment, evaluating breathlessness with and without oxygen, can determine whether oxygen is worth continuing (see 📖 Chapter 5 pp. 76–77).

Non-pharmacological management
- Smoking cessation is important. Individuals with IPF have a 10-fold increased risk of lung cancer regardless of smoking history. This risk is multiplicative with that from continued smoking.
- Pulmonary rehabilitation can improve symptoms such as breathlessness, fatigue, and anxiety, and improve quality of life.
- Referral to a transplant centre may be appropriate in some patients with advanced or progressive disease.

Prognosis
- Median survival is approximately 3 years.
- Severity is best gauged by estimation of the transfer factor (TLCO). Values <40% predicted are indicative of advanced disease.
- A fall in FVC (>10% from baseline) over 6–12 months, or >15% fall in TLCO, are consistent indicators of a poor prognosis.
- Oxygen desaturation during a 6-minute walk test is a strong negative prognostic factor.

NSIP
Corticosteroids, with or without immunosuppressive agents, are the mainstay of treatment. However, the natural progression of disease remains unclear and the optimal regimen, its dose and duration, has not yet been determined.

COP
The cause of COP is unknown. However, the prognosis is good with a prompt response to corticosteroid treatment (prednisolone 0.75–1.0mg/kg). Doses should be weaned over 6–12 months. A longer weaning period or long-term administration is required if patients relapse.

DIP and RB-ILD
These conditions are thought to represent ends of the spectrum of smoking-related ILD with an accumulation of pigmented macrophages seen histologically. Smoking cessation often leads to disease remission. Corticosteroids may be used.

LIP
Corticosteroids are used ± additional immunosuppression. No RCTs exist to guide treatment regimes.

AIP
No single treatment has been of proven benefit. Antibiotics with high-dose corticosteroids (e.g. methylprednisolone 500mg–1g) and supportive measures on an intensive therapy unit are often instigated. The prognosis is poor with an overall mortality of 50%.

Secondary causes of ILD
Data on management are limited with treatment guided towards the underlying cause wherever possible. Corticosteroids ± an immunosuppressive agent are often the mainstay of treatment.

Chest wall and neuromuscular disease

A 55-year-old man with motor neurone disease was referred from the neurology clinic. He complained of early morning headaches and daytime somnolence (he was unable to enjoy watching the television), and was sleeping upright because of orthopnoea. He had bulbar symptoms with a weak voice and dysphagia to solid foods. He was taking riluzole treatment and nutritional supplements. On examination he was thin (BMI 18), tachypnoeic, using his respiratory accessory muscles, and inward movement of the anterior abdominal wall (thoraco-abdominal paradox) was evident on sniffing. His chest was clear. A chest radiograph revealed an elevated left hemidiaphragm, and his vital capacity fell on lying from a standing position (1.82L (34% predicted) to 0.90L). His arterial blood gas (on room air) showed pH 7.39, $PaCO_2$ 8.39, PaO_2 8.61, HCO_3 34.1, BE 12.2.

He was admitted to hospital and nocturnal non-invasive ventilation (NIV) was started. Chest physiotherapy was instigated to aid clearance of secretions and a course of rescue antibiotics provided on discharge for prompt use in case of infection. After 2 months of treatment he reported improvement in his daytime fatigue and concentration, such that he was able to enjoy his favourite television programmes once again.

Respiratory failure is a common terminal event in patients with neuromuscular or chest wall disease. Early recognition and initiation of supportive ventilatory measures has been shown to extend life and provide symptom relief.

Causes
- Pathologies to be considered are shown in Table 1.4.
- Patients with underlying chronic disorders are often under the surveillance of neurology or respiratory specialists. Patients with an unrecognized condition can occasionally present with respiratory failure.

Pathophysiology
During normal sleep many physiological changes occur including:
- Reduced central ventilatory drive.
- Decreased chemoresponsiveness to hypercapnic and hypoxic stimuli.
- Diaphragmatic ventilation accompanying the muscle paralysis that occurs during rapid eye movement (REM) stages.
- Decreased central response to mechanical stimuli (e.g. reduced lung inflation).
- Reduced upper-airway calibre with increased airway resistance.

Table 1.4 Chest wall and neuromuscular causes of chronic respiratory failure

Cause	Examples
Brainstem pathology	Stroke
	Demyelinating disease (multiple sclerosis)
	Arnold-Chiari malformation ± syringobulbia
	Encephalitis
	Space-occupying lesions e.g. tumour
Chest wall deformity	Obesity
	Scoliosis
	Kyphoscoliosis e.g. severe ankylosing spondylitis
	Post trauma/thoracoplasty/sequelae of tuberculosis
Mixed	Polio and post-polio syndrome (PPS—exact mechanism unknown)
	Post ITU ('critical care') neuromyopathy
Myopathy	Acid maltase deficiency
	Duchenne muscular dystrophy
	Myotonic dystrophy
Neuromuscular junction abnormalities	Myasthenia gravis
	Lambert-Eaton myasthenic syndrome (LEMS)
	Botulism
	Organophosphate (anti-cholinesterase) poisoning
Neuropathy	Motor neurone disease (MND)
	Bilateral phrenic nerve palsy
	Guillain Barré syndrome
Spinal cord pathology	Demyelinating disease
	Transverse myelitis
	High cord transection
	Space-occupying lesions e.g. syringomyelia, tumour

In disease states these phenomena may be detrimental. Symptoms may therefore develop as a result of:
- Hypoventilation, which is typically nocturnal (but eventually also during daytime hours). Reasons for this include the following:
  - The central neural stimulus to maintain ventilation, often increased in patients with chest wall or neuromuscular disease, decreases during sleep.
  - Crucial diaphragmatic activity required during REM phases of sleep cannot be achieved in some patients with neuromuscular or chest wall disorders.

- In patients with neuromuscular or chest wall disease, the normal automatic ventilatory response to hypoxia and hypercapnia when awake may be blunted. This worsens during sleep and increases the risk of hypoventilation.
- Inadequate cough and clearance of airway secretions, which increase the risk of sputum retention and pneumonia, especially during concomitant upper respiratory tract infection.

Clinical features

These are often nonspecific and can be mistaken as part of the underlying disease:

- fatigue
- excessive daytime somnolence
- morning headaches
- poor concentration and memory
- exertional dyspnoea
- peripheral oedema
- anorexia.

Paradoxical motion of the diaphragm and abdomen may be evident on examination of the supine patient with diaphragmatic paralysis. An inward movement of the anterior abdominal wall is seen (with loss of the normal synchronized outward motion of both the ribcage and abdomen as the diaphragm descends during inspiration).

Diagnosis

- Spirometry:
  - Supine and erect vital capacity (VC) measures should be included. A reduction in supine VC (>10–20%) is an indirect indicator of diaphragmatic paralysis.
- Arterial blood gases:
  - An increased base excess on a daytime arterial blood gas may be the only evidence of pending ventilatory failure.
  - A compensatory metabolic alkalosis may be seen, i.e. normal pH with $\uparrow PaCO_2$, $\uparrow$base excess, and $\uparrow HCO_3$.
- Overnight oximetry ± transcutaneous CO_2 monitoring:
  - This is a non-invasive surrogate method for continuous measurement of arterial CO_2 tensions.
  - Retention of nocturnal CO_2 with associated hypoxia provides confirmatory evidence of respiratory failure.

Management

- *Respiratory failure:* Nocturnal non-invasive ventilation provides symptom relief and may improve patient survival (see 📖 Chapter 2 pp. 40–42 for practical tips).
- *Optimization of airway secretion clearance:* Respiratory muscle weakness leads to low lung volumes, decreased chest wall compliance, and a weak, ineffective cough. These factors increase the likelihood of recurrent chest infections and secondary damage to the normal mucociliary pathway.

- Physiotherapy advice should be sought early to aid mobilization and expectoration of secretions. Assistance with coughing is often also required.
- Self-assisted strategies, manually assisted strategies, and airway clearance strategies requiring equipment (e.g. mechanical insufflation-exsufflation 'CoughAssist' devices) can all be used and tailored to the patient's needs, either in conjunction with NIPPV or alone.
- These strategies reduce the risk of hospitalization with respiratory complications of the underlying disease and pneumonia.
- *Nutritional status* needs to be optimized.
- *Vigilance for early signs of infection* and prompt treatment is vital.

Pulmonary hypertension

- Pulmonary hypertension (PH) is defined as a mean pulmonary arterial pressure (PAP) of 25mmHg at rest (or >30mmHg with exercise).
- Idiopathic (primary) PH is rare. Secondary PH can complicate many pulmonary, cardiac, and extra-thoracic conditions. Unrelieved pulmonary hypertension, regardless of the cause, leads to right ventricular failure and death.

Causes (World Health Organization Classification, Venice 2003)

Table 1.5 Causes of pulmonary hypertension

1. Pulmonary arterial hypertension	3. Pulmonary hypertension associated with disorders of the respiratory system and/or hypoxaemia
Idiopathic (IPAH; previously known as primary pulmonary hypertension)	
Familial (FPAH)	Chronic obstructive pulmonary disease
Related conditions:	Interstitial lung disease
• Collagen vascular disease (occurs in ~1/3 patients with systemic sclerosis)	Sleep-disordered breathing
	Alveolar hypoventilation disorders
	Chronic exposure to high altitude
• Congenital systemic-to-pulmonary shunts	Developmental abnormalities
• Portal hypertension	**4. Pulmonary hypertension resulting from chronic thrombotic and/or embolic disease**
• HIV infection	
• Drugs/toxins e.g. anorectic agents, rapeseed oil	Thromboembolic obstruction of proximal pulmonary arteries
• Others e.g. thyroid disease, glycogen storage disease, myeloproliferative conditions, sickle cell disease	Thromboembolic obstruction of distal pulmonary arteries
	Non-thrombotic pulmonary embolism (thrombus, tumour, ova and/or parasites, foreign material)
Associated with veno-capillary involvement:	
• Pulmonary veno-occlusive disease	**5. Pulmonary hypertension resulting from miscellaneous disorders**
• Pulmonary capillary haemangiomatosis	
Persistent pulmonary hypertension of the newborn	Inflammatory conditions (e.g. Sarcoidosis, LCH)
	Extrinsic compression of central pulmonary veins: fibrosing mediastinitis, adenopathy, and/or tumours
2. Pulmonary hypertension with left heart disease	
Left-sided atrial or ventricular heart disease	
Left-sided valvular heart disease	

Clinical features

Symptoms are often nonspecific and develop insidiously.
- Common:
  - Exertional dyspnoea, fatigue.
  - Exertional chest pain, syncope, peripheral oedema (right ventricular failure) in more advanced disease.

- Less common:
  - Haemoptysis, cough, Ortner's syndrome (rare, hoarseness due to left recurrent laryngeal nerve compression by a dilated main pulmonary artery).

Investigations

The following investigations can establish the diagnosis of PH, elicit any underlying cause, and determine the effect on cardio-respiratory function. CXR and ECG are abnormal in over 85% of patients.

- CXR:
  - Characteristically shows prominent pulmonary arteries ± peripheral vessel attenuation, resulting in oligaemic lung fields. Underlying lung disease may be evident.
- ECG:
  - Often reveals right ventricular hypertrophy or strain.
- Echocardiography is the most useful non-invasive diagnostic test:
  - Identifies right heart enlargement. Tricuspid regurgitation may be seen, and from this the pulmonary artery systolic pressure can be estimated non-invasively using Doppler techniques. Right ventricular dilatation and hypertrophy are late findings.
- Right heart cardiac catheterization:
  - Remains the gold standard for a definitive diagnosis and accurate determination of the PAP.

The following tests can help elicit a potential underlying cause:
- Pulmonary function testing:
  - Can quantify the severity of underlying restrictive or obstructive lung disease.
- Arterial blood gases ± overnight oximetry:
  - PH may develop consequent to transient oxygen desaturation, and normal resting daytime oxygen saturation does not exclude exertional or nocturnal hypoxia.
- Ventilation/Perfusion (V/Q) scan or CTPA:
  - To exclude chronic thromboembolism.
- High resolution CT scanning:
  - To exclude parenchymal lung disease.

Treatment

General measures include:
- Oxygen therapy should be considered for all hypoxic patients. Hypoxaemia exerts a pulmonary vasoconstrictive effect and supplementation should aim to maintain an oxygen saturation >90%.
- Diuretics should be used if there is evidence of peripheral oedema secondary to right heart failure. A low dose, e.g. spironolactone 25mg or furosemide 40mg daily, should be initiated with close monitoring to avoid excessive diuresis and renal impairment.
- Digoxin is a positive inotrope and has produced favourable acute haemodynamic effects in patients with right ventricular failure and primary pulmonary hypertension. Low doses of 125mcg daily are often sufficient. Long-term effects and impact on patient mortality are unknown.
- Tailored exercise training may have a role.

- Contraceptive advice is necessary for patients of child-bearing age. Pregnancy and PPH is associated with a maternal mortality rate of 30–50% as a consequence of the increased demand on the maternal cardiopulmonary system.
- Annual influenza immunizations and pneumococcal vaccination are needed.

Idiopathic (primary) PH

- Treatment is complex and patients should be referred to a specialist centre (in the UK: Cambridge, Glasgow, London (Hammersmith), Newcastle, Sheffield).
- Anticoagulation has been shown to improve prognosis in PPH, and lifelong warfarin therapy (aiming for an international normalized ratio (INR) of 2) is recommended. The precise reason for the benefits seen remains unclear.
- Calcium channel antagonists are used in ~20% of patients with a positive acute vasoreactivity test response (administration of a short-acting vasodilator induces a mean pulmonary artery pressure decrease of at least 10mmHg). If there is no clinical response after 3–6 months advanced treatment should be initiated.
- Advanced therapies include:
  - Prostaglandin analogues e.g. continuous intravenous epoprostenol infusion, continuous subcutaneous or intravenous treprostinil infusion, inhaled iloprost.
  - Endothelin receptor antagonists e.g. bosentan.
  - Nitric oxide.
  - Phosphodiesterase (PDE) inhibitors e.g. sildenafil.
- The role of combination therapy is not yet fully established.
- Atrial septostomy and lung transplantation are reserved for patients refractory to medical therapy.

Secondary PH

- Stop precipitating medication/toxin exposure.
- Optimize management of underlying condition.
- Reverse hypoxia (hypoxaemia is a potent pulmonary vasoconstrictor).
- Consider anti-retrovirals in HIV-related PH.

Referral for specialist evaluation should be made if PH persists despite aggressive conventional management. Prostaglandin analogues, sildenafil, and nitric oxide may reduce pulmonary vascular resistance but their role in secondary PH is not yet clear.

Chronic thromboembolic pulmonary hypertension (CTEPH)
- CTEPH occurs in up to 3.8% of patients at 2 years after an acute pulmonary embolism.
- Thromboendarterectomy for accessible (main, lobar, or segmental arteries) chronic thrombi is potentially curative. The peri-operative mortality is <5% when used for selected patients in specialist centres.
- All patients are maintained on lifelong anticoagulation.

Prognosis
Idiopathic (primary) PH
- The median estimated survival following diagnosis is 2.8y, with 5y survival rates of approximately 34%.
- Patients without significant right ventricular dysfunction and responders to the newer therapies may survive >10 years.

Factors associated with a poor prognosis include:
- Functional: New York Heart Association (NYHA) class III or IV; poor 6-minute walk distance.
- Echocardiographic: presence of a pericardial effusion or large right atrium.
- Haemodynamic: significantly elevated right atrial pressure or mean pulmonary arterial pressure at presentation; reduced cardiac index.
- Demographic: longer time from symptom onset to diagnosis; age >45 years.
- Other: lack of therapeutic response to prostaglandin analogue after 3–6 months; increased serum N-terminal prohormone brain natriuretic peptide (NT-proBNP) levels; right ventricular hypertrophy on ECG.

Secondary PH
Prognosis depends on severity of the underlying disease and degree of right ventricular impairment.

Cystic fibrosis

- Cystic fibrosis is the most common fatal inherited disease in European populations (incidence 1 in 2500 births, carrier frequency 1:25).
- It is an autosomal recessive disease, with inheritance of a mutation of the gene encoding the cystic fibrosis transmembrane conductance regulator protein (CFTR)—a cyclic-AMP regulated chloride channel. This defect prevents normal transmembrane salt and water movement, resulting in viscous intra-luminal (e.g. airway) secretions.
- Irreversible bronchiectasis occurs as a consequence of reduced mucociliary clearance of thickened secretions, secondary bacterial colonization, and resultant inflammation.
- Pancreatic insufficiency often develops as the exocrine ducts become plugged by viscid secretions. This leads to pancreatic enzyme insufficiency with resultant malabsorption, and progressive pancreatic destruction/fibrosis.
- Over 600 different mutations exist, the most common of which is the delta F 508 (ΔF508), which affects about 67% of patients.
- In the UK, neonates are screened with a heel-prick test for immunoreactive trypsin (IRT).
- Patient management often moves from the paediatric to adult setting aged 16–18 years.

Diagnosis

Patients are usually diagnosed as a child/neonate with confirmatory genetic/biochemical tests. Diagnosis in adulthood is associated with different alleles and a milder phenotype.

Management

A multidisciplinary approach is necessary, with shared care from a variety of specialists: respiratory physician, clinical nurse specialist, physiotherapist, dietician, pharmacist, and psychologist. Gastroenterology and endocrinology expertise may also be required.

Lung disease

- Minimizing infection:
  - Regular chest physiotherapy: airway clearance techniques and exercise.
  - Prompt use of appropriate antibiotics (often requires higher doses and longer courses).
  - Monitoring sputum for organisms i.e. *Pseudomonas aeruginosa*, *Burkholderia cepacia*.
- Maintaining pulmonary function:
  - Bronchodilators and corticosteroids (inhaled or oral) may be helpful, particularly if there is concomitant asthma.
- Early consideration of assessment for transplantation.

Nutritional

- Optimization of calorie intake:
  - Malnutrition directly correlates with poor lung function and prognosis.

- High calorie intake is advised aiming to achieve a BMI >20.
- Nasogastric tube or gastrostomy feeding may be required.
- Adequate pancreatic enzyme supplementation.

Gastrointestinal
- Screen annually for cirrhosis/portal hypertension.

Endocrine
- Screen annually for diabetes, as symptomatic disease is often preceded by a period of impaired glucose tolerance. Insulin therapy is usually required to achieve glycaemic control.
- Preventive measures to minimize CF-related osteoporosis include improving dietary calcium intake, increasing physical activity, and adequate vitamin D, K, and calcium supplementation if required.

Fertility
- Males are infertile with >98% having obstructive azoospermia. Females are usually subfertile.

Psychological
- Aid development of coping strategies for dealing with progressive life-limiting disease.
- Encourage adoption of normal routine (e.g. education, employment etc.).
- Address underlying depression, anxiety, and emotional difficulties.
- Support through pre-transplant assessment, bereavement counselling, and end of life decision-making.

Prognosis
The predicted life expectancy of a person diagnosed with CF at birth is approximately 42 years. The main causes of death are respiratory, including chronic respiratory failure, infection, and massive haemoptysis.

Further reading

American Thoracic Society/European Respiratory Society (2002) American Thoracic Society/European Respiratory Society international multidisciplinary consensus classification of the idiopathic interstitial pneumonias. *Am J Respir Crit Care Med*; 165: 277–304.

Annane D, Orlikowski D, Chevret S, Chevrolet JC, Raphaël JC (2007) Nocturnal mechanical ventilation for chronic hypoventilation in patients with neuromuscular and chest wall disorders. *Cochrane Database Syst Rev*; Oct 17; (4): CD001941.

Bradley B, Branley HM, Egan JJ, *et al.* (2008) Interstitial lung disease guideline: British Thoracic Society Interstitial Lung Disease guideline group. *Thorax*; 63 (Suppl 5): 1–58.

British Thoracic Society (2006) *The burden of lung disease, 2nd edition*. http://www.erpho.org.uk/Download/Public/15381/1/BurdenLungDisease2006.pdf.

Cystic Fibrosis Foundation website (USA): www.cff.org.

Cystic Fibrosis Trust website (UK): www.cftrust.org.uk.

Goldstraw P, Crowley J, Chansky K, *et al.* (2007) The IASLC Lung Cancer Staging Project: Proposals for the revision of the TNM stage groups in the forthcoming (seventh) edition of the TNM classification of malignant tumours. *J Thorac Oncol*; 2: 706.

Lababede O, Meziane MA, Rice TW (1999) TNM staging of lung cancer: A quick reference chart. *Chest*; 115: 233–235.

Murray SA, Kendall M, Boyd K, Sheikh A (2005) Clinical review: Illness trajectories and palliative care. *BMJ*; 330: 1007–1011.

National Collaborating Centre for Chronic Conditions (2004) Chronic obstructive pulmonary disease. National clinical guideline on management of chronic obstructive pulmonary disease in adults in primary and secondary care. *Thorax*; 59 (Suppl 1): 1–232.

National Pulmonary Hypertension Centres of the UK and Ireland (2008) Consensus statement on the management of pulmonary hypertension in clinical practice in the UK and Ireland. *Thorax*; 63 (Suppl 2): 1–41.

Robinson BWS, Musk AW, Lake RA (2005) Seminar: Malignant mesothelioma. *Lancet*; 366: 397–408.

Chapter 2

Chronic respiratory failure from end-stage disease

Definition

Respiratory failure is defined as the presence of hypoxaemia (PaO_2 <8kPa) with or without hypercapnia ($PaCO_2$ >6.0kPa). It is divided into two types:

- Type I:
  - Hypoxaemia with normal or low CO_2.
  - Typically a result of inadequate pulmonary gas exchange (raised alveolar-to-arterial, A-a, gradient).
- Type II:
  - Hypoxaemia with an increased $PaCO_2$.
  - Usually a consequence of hypoventilation ± V/Q mismatching.
  - Chronicity indicated by an elevated base excess and bicarbonate, to maintain normal serum pH (metabolic alkalosis due to renal compensation for high $PaCO_2$).

Pathophysiology

Chronic respiratory failure can arise from an abnormality in any of the components of ventilatory control, including the central or peripheral nervous systems, respiratory muscle, chest wall, airways, or alveoli. It may be classified as:

- Failure of ventilatory drive e.g. brainstem stroke, iatrogenic suppression (e.g. opioids).
- Respiratory pump failure e.g. neuropathy, myopathy (see 📖 Chapter 1 pp. 22–25).
- Neuromuscular junction pathology.
- Chest wall deformity/restriction e.g. scoliosis, obesity.
- Obstructive lung pathology e.g. airways obstruction (COPD, chronic asthma), obliterative bronchiolitis.
- Mixed e.g. obstructive sleep apnoea (OSA) combined with obesity-related hypoventilation; OSA in a patient with COPD; post-ITU ('critical care') neuromyopathy.

Determining the underlying cause(s) is fundamental to guiding optimal therapy.

Hypoxaemia is often the potent stimulus of respiratory drive for patients with chronic respiratory failure. Administration of high concentrations of supplemental oxygen can suppress this drive and result in acute respiratory acidosis ($\uparrow\uparrow PaCO_2$) and decompensation of an otherwise stable state.

Clinical features

Chronic respiratory failure will often develop as a result of previously diagnosed disease after years of illness. An early appreciation of this risk can help to pre-empt difficult future management decisions. In patients who present *de novo* following good health, investigations and treatment must run concurrently to identify co-morbid and reversible causes of deterioration. The tests below must therefore be performed with this in mind and are indicated only when they would alter patients' management.

Symptoms
- Dyspnoea:
  - on exertion (although may be masked in patients with muscle weakness and limited mobility)
  - orthopnoea
  - dyspnoea whilst swimming (typically associated with diaphragmatic weakness).
- Fatigue.
- Reduced appetite.
- Symptoms from chronic nocturnal hypoventilation:
  - excessive daytime sleepiness
  - headache/confusion on awakening
  - poor concentration
  - sleep disturbance/nightmares.
- Anxiety.
- Recurrent chest infections:
  - These occur often as a consequence of aspiration secondary to laryngeal and/or pharyngeal weakness.
- Peripheral oedema:
  - Particularly in COPD, the effect of hypoxia may result in fluid retention (cor pulmonale).

Symptoms typically develop over a prolonged period of time, occasionally years. Given the insidious onset, clues are often missed or attributed to underlying disease progression. Concurrent, occasionally innocuous, illness may precipitate decompensation of long-standing respiratory failure. Acute respiratory failure with development of hypercapnia may result in confusion, reduced level of consciousness, or coma.

Examination
- Signs of respiratory failure:
  - General: increased respiratory effort i.e. tachypnoea, prominent use of accessory respiratory muscles.
  - Hypoxia: central cyanosis, polycythaemia, fluid retention, cor pulmonale.
  - Hypercapnia: bounding pulse, tremor/flap, papilloedema, drowsiness, confusion.
- Full neurological assessment may reveal signs of a known, or undiagnosed, neuromuscular condition e.g. fasciculation, muscle wasting, myotonia, and weakness.

- Diaphragmatic weakness may be revealed by paradoxical thoraco-abdominal movement (inward movement of the abdominal wall during inspiration).

Investigations

Arterial blood gases

- A raised $PaCO_2$ ($PaCO_2$ >6.0kPa) is indicative of chronic type II respiratory failure.
- An elevated base excess (>+2mmol/L) ± high bicarbonate (>28mmol/L) indicates chronicity of respiratory failure.
- The alveolar to arterial (A-a) gradient is usually raised (>2–3kPa) when V/Q mismatch is present, i.e. abnormal lung parenchyma, but normal with underlying central or neuromyopathic disease.

Imaging

- A CXR may show features of airway obstruction or a complication of the underlying disease e.g. pneumonia or pneumothorax.
- CT/MRI brain imaging can reveal presence of an underlying stroke or tumour.

Pulmonary function tests

- Reveal extent of airflow obstruction or restriction.
- Determine vital capacity.
- Assess diaphragm/respiratory muscle weakness e.g. discrepancy between lying and standing vital capacity.

Others

- A sleep study may reveal features of obstructive sleep apnoea and nocturnal hypoxia e.g. in obesity-related hypoventilation.
- An EMG should be considered if an underlying myopathy or MND is suspected. Subsequent muscle biopsy may be required.
- Blood tests may provide useful information e.g. acetylcholine receptor antibodies detected in cases of suspected myasthenia gravis, or elevated creatine kinase concentrations in some myopathies.

Oxygen therapy in chronic respiratory failure

Most data supporting the use of oxygen in chronic respiratory failure stem from patients with COPD. There is little evidence guiding its application in other disease states, and the research base underpinning oxygen use in dyspnoea palliation is scanty (see 📖 Chapter 5 pp. 76–77). No reliable factors predict which patients will benefit from oxygen therapy and medical management of all underlying conditions must be optimized prior to its consideration.

Types of oxygen therapy

Ambulatory oxygen

- This is delivered by a portable, lightweight cylinder and used during exercise/daily activities.
- Ambulatory oxygen may be considered for:
  - mobile patients on LTOT
  - patients who experience improvement in exercise tolerance ± dyspnoea with oxygen supplementation.

Short-burst oxygen therapy (SBOT)

- SBOT involves intermittent use of oxygen at rest, prior to exertion, during exercise (ambulatory oxygen), or during recovery.
- There is some evidence that use of oxygen during exercise can improve exercise capacity and breathlessness in patients with COPD. Systematic reviews of clinical trials suggest that oxygen at rest is not usually effective at relieving symptoms.
- No factors predict which patients will benefit; therefore, individual therapeutic trials with clinical assessment of subjective gains may be appropriate.
- This topic is considered in further detail in 📖 Chapter 5 pp. 76–77.

Long-term oxygen therapy (LTOT)

COPD patients

- Landmark trials[1,2] have shown that LTOT, administered for ≥15hrs/d (including when asleep), increases survival and quality of life in patients with hypoxaemic COPD. A greater benefit may be gained from application of oxygen for >19hrs/d.
- Further studies have demonstrated improvement in cardiovascular morbidity, sleep quality, secondary polycythaemia, neuropsychological and cognitive function, exercise capacity, sleep quality, and frequency of hospitalization.
- Peripheral oedema due to cor pulmonale is reduced as reversal of hypoxaemia improves renal perfusion and increases salt/water excretion.
- LTOT does not influence the decline in FEV1.
- Current indications for LTOT in COPD patients:
  - PaO_2 <7.3kPa breathing room air when clinically stable.

- PaO$_2$ >7.3 kPa but <8kPa when clinically stable with one of: secondary polycythaemia; nocturnal hypoxaemia (SaO$_2$ <90% for >30% of the night); peripheral oedema; or pulmonary hypertension.
- Assessment should comprise arterial blood gas (ABG) measurements on two occasions at least 4 weeks apart in patients who are receiving optimum medical management and whose COPD is stable (ideally >6 weeks following an exacerbation).
- Arterial hypoxaemia in COPD patients with a FEV1 >40% or 1.5L suggests that there may be another cause (e.g. pulmonary emboli or nocturnal hypoventilation) and further investigations are appropriate.

Non-COPD patients
- Evidence is limited. Use of LTOT in patients with chronic hypoxaemia related to other pulmonary or non-pulmonary conditions (i.e. interstitial lung disease, terminal cancer, or chronic heart failure) has not been shown to improve survival.

Practical applications

- Nasal cannulae or a face mask may be used.
- An oxygen flow rate of 2–4L/min is often initiated, but controlled concentration oxygen (24% or 28%) may be given via a mask.
- Aim for an oxygen saturation 90–92% (PaO$_2$ 8–9kPa).
- Check ABG on LTOT to assess for hypercapnia, especially if raised PaCO$_2$ at baseline or if patient develops suggestive symptoms e.g. morning headache, daytime somnolence.
- Although smoking is considered a contraindication to oxygen use, many patients continue to smoke. They must be warned about the flammability risks and probably negated benefit from treatment.
- Oxygen concentrators are the most efficient source of LTOT and can deliver up to 10L/min of oxygen. Multiple concentrators may be joined using a Y-shaped adapter to allow a higher flow if required.

References

1. Nocturnal Oxygen Therapy Trial Group (1980) Continuous or nocturnal oxygen therapy in hypoxemic chronic obstructive lung disease: a clinical trial. *Ann Intern Med*; 93: 391–398.
2. Medical Research Council Working Party (1981) Long-term domiciliary oxygen therapy in chronic hypoxic cor pulmonale complicating chronic bronchitis and emphysema. *Lancet*; 1: 681–686.

Non-invasive ventilation in chronic respiratory failure

Non-invasive ventilation (NIV) has an important role in the management of patients with chronic hypercapnic respiratory failure. However, there are no data to suggest that prophylactic NIV is beneficial for patients at risk of developing chronic respiratory failure and it is not a substitute for invasive ventilation in patients for whom escalation of treatment, i.e. intubation, is appropriate.

Indications
Deciding when to start NIV will differ between patients. Potential clinical benefits, such as relief of morning headaches and reduced daytime sleepiness, should be balanced with patient wishes and ability to tolerate the intervention.
- NIV should be considered in patients with symptomatic chronic hypercapnic respiratory failure, and/or evidence of nocturnal hypoventilation on overnight oximetry.
- Common underlying conditions include:
  - neuromuscular weakness e.g. muscular dystrophies, myopathy
  - thoracic wall deformity
  - decompensated obstructive sleep apnoea
  - obesity hypoventilation syndrome.
- Development of respiratory failure in MND/ALS occurs with advanced disease and often results in frightening dyspnoea (~85% patients). NIV has been shown to improve survival and quality of life, and reduce sleep disruption (less REM sleep). It does not influence respiratory muscle weakness or disease progression.
- The role of NIV in patients with severe COPD and chronic hypercapnic respiratory failure remains unclear. There are reports of it being used very near the end of life to palliate breathlessness when other measures are ineffective or cause adverse effects, or in order to 'buy time' to organize affairs or await the arrival of family (see box on p. 42).
- In patients with cystic fibrosis and progressive respiratory failure, nocturnal NIV may be required, to act as a 'bridge' to transplantation.

Contraindications
NIV is contraindicated or should be used with caution in the following situations. As always, the balance of potential benefits and burdens should be weighed up in each individual patient.
- Inability to use mask: facial trauma/surgery/deformity.
- Inability to protect the airway: moderate to severe bulbar impairment/impaired mental status/agitation/upper airway obstruction.
- Excessive respiratory secretions.
- Vomiting/recent oesophageal surgery or injury.
- Haemodynamic instability e.g. cardiac arrhythmia.
- Untreated pneumothorax.
- Life-threatening refractory hypoxaemia.

Practical applications

Although NIV is usually administered nocturnally, control of daytime symptoms is seen. This is likely to be from a combined effect of relief of muscle fatigue, improved chest wall compliance, and reversal of nocturnal hypoventilation.

Ventilator

A portable non-invasive positive pressure ventilator (NIPPV) is used in most cases. If this is not tolerated a negative pressure ventilator (i.e. iron lung), abdominal ventilator, or rocking bed device may be tried.

Interface

Nasal masks are preferred by the majority of patients. Alternatives include oro-nasal masks or a mouthpiece.

Compliance

Patients may find it difficult to tolerate the ventilator, and a failure to respond clinically may reflect non-compliance. Equipment adjustments are often necessary i.e. ventilation settings, mask size or type, and strap tension. A humidifier can be added if mucosal dryness is troublesome. Most patients adapt within weeks and this is enhanced if symptomatic improvement has been noticed (often seen with ≥4hrs NIV use each night).

Monitoring

Patient compliance, symptom response, and features suggestive of hypercapnia should be noted. Repeat nocturnal studies for patients using NIV are usually required only if there is failure to improve or deterioration (with no obvious clinical precedent).

Withdrawal of NIV

Deterioration in respiratory function with increased dependency on ventilatory support (i.e. daytime NIV use) is inevitable in the majority of patients with neuromuscular disease who initiate NIV. Recurrence of previously controlled symptoms, i.e. morning headaches, and progression of the patient's underlying disease despite escalation of ventilatory support (i.e. higher inspiratory pressure settings) indicate insipient failure of ventilatory control. Preparation for this, at its instigation, is important. Good, early communication can avoid distress when clinical decline occurs.

A structured plan should be clearly documented prior to treatment, stating the patient's suitability for future invasive mechanical ventilation. This may be in the form of a statement of wishes or preferences, or an advance decision, and should be informed by medical opinion (see 📖 Chapter 8 pp. 174–176).

All patients should be able to opt to discontinue supportive therapy at any point regardless of clinical status. Practical steps involved in the withdrawal of NIV are described in 📖 Chapter 12 pp. 262–263.

Mrs O was 37 years old and dying of lung cancer. She was a single parent, living alone with a 7-year-old daughter, Amy, and was divorced and estranged from her daughter's father. Her mother was alive and well and helped to care for Amy at times, although she also worked.

Mrs O had a respiratory infection requiring admission to hospital. She wanted to be ventilated, but as she had bony metastases and rib fracture this was not possible. However, she received NIV on the ward and made a partial recovery. She then quickly asked for and chaired a case conference, and organized care for her daughter in the event of her death. She also spent a weekend at home for Amy's birthday.

Shortly after returning to hospital she developed another infection and this time refused intervention. A paper detailing the discussion and decisions made at the case conference was put into a memory box for Amy, to show her how much her mother cared for her.

Chapter 3

Health-related quality of life in end-stage respiratory disease

Causes of poor health-related quality of life

There is indisputable evidence that patients with advanced respiratory disease experience a poor quality of life. Studies show that the majority of such patients describe their quality of life as only 'fair' or 'poor'.

Importantly, the quality of life of patients with non-malignant chronic respiratory disease (CRD) is at least as poor as that of patients with advanced cancer, and a number of studies have shown that it may, indeed, be even worse. The disease trajectory in CRD starts and continues at a lower functional level than that of patients with malignant disease (see 📖 Chapter 1 pp. 4–5), and tends to last longer. In other words, patients with CRD may have to cope with a worse quality of life for longer than those with cancer.

A wide range of health-related factors impact on patients' quality of life, including uncontrolled symptoms and unmet social, practical, psychological, communication, and education needs.

Symptoms

The symptom burden experienced by those with advanced respiratory disease is considerable. In both chronic respiratory disease and lung cancer, the mean number of symptoms per patient is seven.

Table 3.1 documents the approximate prevalence of symptoms in patients with benign and malignant advanced respiratory disease. The wide range of prevalence data reflects the heterogeneity of study populations and outcome measures. Patients with lung cancer develop more pain, anorexia, and constipation, whereas those with CRD suffer more breathlessness, anxiety, and depression. Many of these symptoms are never adequately controlled. There is evidence that patients with CRD are less likely to receive symptom control interventions than those with lung cancer or other malignant disease.

Psychosocial needs

Approximately 40% of patients with advanced COPD are largely house-bound, leaving the house less than once a month. Despite this, there is a significant lack of home-based services, with only 13% of patients seeing a nurse regularly at home.[1]

Studies have shown that patients with advanced respiratory disease suffer extensive unmet psychological and social needs:
- Patients are often socially isolated. Breathlessness hinders movement from the home. Those with advanced CRD tend to be particularly isolated and have been described as 'socially invisible'. Such patients tend to have a lower socioeconomic status, which further restricts external activities and access to help.
- Patients suffer considerable psychological morbidity, with anxiety and low mood being highly prevalent (see 📖 Chapter 6 pp. 116–121).

- Patients' information requirements are not matched by what they receive. Those with CRD appear to have particularly great information and education needs. They wish to know about disease self-management, prognosis, and the existence of social and financial help.
- Care-givers have great demands placed upon them, and yet are rarely given support themselves. They experience significant morbidity as a result.

Table 3.1 Symptom prevalence in advanced COPD and lung cancer

Symptom	COPD (%)	Lung cancer (%)
Fatigue	70–95	50–60
Breathlessness	60–95	45–75
Cough	60–80	30–80
Insomnia	55–75	10–60
Anxiety	30–75	10–45
Pain	20–80	50–90
Depression	15–75	15–70
Anorexia	10–80	35–75
Constipation	25–45	30–60
Nausea	5–45	15–45

Reference

1. Elkington H, White P, Addington-Hall J, et al. (2005) The healthcare needs of chronic obstructive pulmonary disease patients in the last year of life. *Palliat Med*; 19: 485–491.

Barriers to provision of care

The most fundamental barrier to the provision of good end of life care is failure to recognize the approach of the end of life.

Patients with advanced respiratory disease experience significant physical and psychological morbidity (see Table 3.1). In order to improve the care provided to these patients, it is important to understand the factors that hinder the provision of adequate care.

Prognostication difficulties

Prognosticating is notoriously difficult in all advanced disease. It is a particular challenge in patients with CRD, or lung cancer with underlying CRD, because of the unpredictable disease trajectory (see 📖 Chapter 1 pp. 4–5). Slow functional decline is punctuated by periods of acute decline, which occur unpredictably. Death tends to occur during one of these episodes and, again, it is hard to predict during which episode this may happen.

It is not easy to provide care that meets the end of life needs of a patient when it has not yet been considered that a patient may be approaching the end of life.

Communication challenges

Exacerbations causing respiratory failure (particularly in patients with CRD) occur suddenly and unpredictably, and the outcome is often determined by last-minute decisions regarding life support. It is usually only possible to discover patients' end of life preferences if these have been established in advance (see 📖 Chapter 8 pp. 174–176). Such advance care planning is often inadequate, making it harder to conform to patients' wishes and provide appropriate end of life care.

Misconceptions about respiratory disease

Although the poor prognosis of patients with advanced lung cancer is fully appreciated, patients and their carers generally fail to understand that CRD is a life-threatening, progressive disease that causes an inexorable decline in health status and function. Good end of life care is impossible without recognition that death may occur prematurely.

Furthermore, the appreciation amongst patients who have smoked that their disease is to some extent self-inflicted leads some patients to believe that they are not eligible for, or deserving of, measures to improve their quality of life.

Misconceptions about end of life care

In the 'death-denying culture' pervasive in many 'developed' countries, embarking on care that acknowledges the approach of the end of life can be misconstrued as evidence of failure or 'giving up'. Patients and professionals often still expect a dichotomous model of care moving from disease modification to palliation, despite this now having been superceded by a mixed model of care combining both approaches (see 📖 Chapter 10 p. 214).

Resource limitations

Resource limitations form a significant impediment to the delivery of effective end of life care. Even for cancer patients (the historical focus of good end of life care) provision of care is not uniform and patients' needs are not always met.

Improving care for all patients with advanced respiratory disease has significant funding and manpower implications. Specialists in end of life care (specialist palliative care) are not always well informed about the management of non-malignant respiratory disease, and respiratory specialists may lack skills in the palliation of symptoms and provision of end of life care.

Lack of research evidence

Research involving vulnerable patients with advanced disease is beset by significant ethical and methodological challenges. These include difficulties in gaining informed consent, poor recruitment rates, and high attrition rates. The lack of evidence to support patient management greatly hinders the provision of high quality end of life care.

Further reading

Claessens MT, Lynn J, Zhong Z, et al. (2000) Dying with lung cancer or chronic obstructive pulmonary disease: insights from SUPPORT Study to Understand Prognoses and Preferences for Outcomes and Risks of Treatments. *J Am Geriatr Soc;* 48: S146–153.

Habraken J, Riet G, Gore JJ et al. (2009) Health-related quality of life in end-stage COPD and lung cancer patients. *J Pain Sy Manage;* 37 (6): 973–981.

Skilbeck J, Mott L, Page H, et al. (1998) Palliative care in chronic obstructive airways disease: a needs assessment. *Palliat Med;* 12: 245–254.

Spathis A, Booth S. (2008) End of life care in chronic obstructive pulmonary disease. *International Journal of COPD;* 3 (1): 11–29.

Chapter 4

Recognizing the end of life phase

Definitions

'The art of living well and dying well are one.'

Epicurus

End of life care, palliative care, supportive care, and terminal care are terms that many use interchangeably. There are, as yet, no internationally agreed definitions that explicitly describe the differences between each type of care, greatly hindering the accurate use and full understanding of these terms. For the purposes of this handbook, the following definitions are used.

End of life care

End of life care helps all those with advanced, progressive, incurable illness to live as well as possible until they die. It enables the supportive and palliative care needs of both patient and family to be identified and met throughout the last phase of life and into bereavement. It includes the management of pain and other symptoms and provision of psychological, social, spiritual, and practical support. End of life care is underpinned by:

• An active and compassionate approach to care that ensures respect for and dignity of the patient and family.
• Partnership in care between patient, family, and health and social care professionals.
• Regular and systematic assessment of patient/carer needs incorporating patient consent at all times.
• Anticipation and management of deterioration in the patient's state of health and well-being.
• Advance care planning in accordance with patient preferences.
• Patient choice about place of care and death.
• Sensitivity to personal, cultural, and spiritual beliefs and practices.
• Effective coordination of care across all teams and providers of care.

There is no consensus as to the definition of the beginning of end of life care. Many consider that the end of life phase has started when a person with advanced, progressive disease could have a prognosis of less than one year. However, others relate the start of end of life care to when a patient develops palliative care needs, for example requiring control of symptoms and/or psychosocial support.

Palliative care and supportive care

Both terms are well represented by the definition of end of life care above. Arguably, the main difference between end of life care and palliative or supportive care is that the latter is provided from the time of diagnosis with incurable, progressive disease, irrespective of the length of prognosis, whereas end of life care has been arbitrarily defined as occurring within approximately one year of the time of death.

Although the terms palliative care and supportive care are largely used interchangeably, there are some subtle differences between them:

- Supportive care is an 'umbrella term' that encompasses a broad range of services that can help support patients, without being directed at treating the illness itself. This would include self-help, information giving, social support, and rehabilitation, and does also incorporate palliative care. Although palliative care practitioners would often provide such support, supportive care is arguably a broader construct than palliative care.
- Supportive care is given to any patient with a chronic disease, even if the disease does not impact on length of life. For example, patients with cancer who are treated and cured may still require supportive care.
- Palliative care has evolved into a distinct specialty, with associated specialist training. Supportive care, however, is like generalist palliative care, and its provision is the responsibility of all healthcare professionals.

Generalist palliative care

Generalist palliative care is a vital and routine part of clinical practice that aims to promote physical and psychological health, regardless of diagnosis or prognosis.

All healthcare professionals who look after patients with incurable, progressive disease are providing generalist palliative care. The vast majority of palliative care is provided by patients' own healthcare teams, and does not need to be provided by palliative care specialists. It is a duty and a privilege for all healthcare professionals to be able to provide compassionate and effective care from diagnosis to death.

Specialist palliative care

Specialist palliative care is provided by teams that specialize in providing palliative care for patients with particularly complex needs, including uncontrolled intractable symptoms and complex psychosocial needs.

Specialist palliative care became a medical specialty in the UK in 1987. Care is provided by specialist teams trained in the art and science of palliative care with extensive experience in providing symptom control and psychosocial/spiritual support for patients with complex needs. Referral criteria for specialist palliative care are given in 📖 Chapter 10 p. 220, and include care of patients with uncontrolled, intractable symptoms or complex psychosocial issues.

Specialist palliative care developed in response to the needs of patients with cancer, and in most countries care is still mainly provided for patients with malignant disease. However, there is increasing recognition that specialist palliative care must be provided to patients based on need rather than diagnosis.

Terminal care

Terminal care refers to the care that is provided to patients who only have a few days or hours to live (see 📖 Chapter 12).

Prognostication

It is not possible to provide high quality end of life care if it is not yet recognized that the end of life is, indeed, approaching. This section considers factors that can be used to help predict prognosis. Practical measures for determining and communicating prognosis are considered in detail in 📖 Chapter 8 pp. 172–173.

Prediction of prognosis

Predicting prognosis is notoriously hard. Doctors tend to be over-optimistic in predicting prognosis. According to a large cohort study,[1] doctors only make an accurate prognosis 20% of the time, and overestimate the prognosis of patients with incurable disease by a factor of five.

More experienced doctors tend to be more accurate. However, the better the doctor knows the patient and the more recent the last contact with the patient, the less accurate the prediction of prognosis. Anecdotally, patients prognosticate more accurately than healthcare professionals, and those that verbalize suspicion of a short prognosis are often correct.

Predicting prognosis relies on an understanding of typical disease trajectories (see 📖 Chapter 1 pp. 4–5). The principle differences between the trajectory for cancer (a) and COPD (b) are:

- The cancer trajectory is shorter with relatively good functioning until the last few months. The COPD trajectory involves a lower level of functioning for a more prolonged time.
- Patients with cancer tend to deteriorate rapidly in the last few weeks or months of life and the prognosis tends to be relatively predictable. The prognosis of those with COPD is hard to predict, as death may occur during any one of the many acute exacerbations.

Malignant disease

The prognosis of patients with malignant lung disease is very poor, usually measured in months from the time of diagnosis. The prediction of prognosis is made easier by this, and by the fact that the disease trajectory tends to involve an exponential decline. Initially deterioration in condition is seen month by month, then week by week and, in the terminal phase, day by day.

In practice in malignant disease, a pragmatic and useful way of predicting prognosis is to find out how quickly a patient's condition is changing. If it is changing month by month, the prognosis tends to be measured in a few months, if week by week, then a few weeks, and if day by day, then a few days.

Non-malignant disease

Prognostication is particularly challenging in patients with advanced non-malignant respiratory disease, because of the relatively lengthy deterioration and the fact that death occurs unpredictably during one of the many acute short-lived exacerbations of disease.

Many prognostication tools have been developed to try to integrate the various factors that impact on prognosis. In advanced COPD, the most commonly used is the BODE index, which generates a score out of 10, based on body mass index, degree of airflow obstruction, dyspnoea score, and exercise capacity. A score of 7 or more gives a 4-year survival of only 20%. However, in practice this index is not particularly useful in determining which patients are likely to die in the next year (see Table 4.1).

A number of other clinical indicators can alert professionals to a prognosis of less than a year. The degree of dyspnoea has been shown to be a more reliable indicator of both a poor prognosis and a willingness to discuss end of life issues than disease severity or pulmonary function:

• MRC grade 4/5 i.e. shortness of breath after 100m on the level or confined to the house because of breathlessness.
• More than three admissions in 12 months with COPD exacerbations.
• Disease assessed to be severe (e.g. FEV1 <30% predicted in patients with COPD).
• Fulfillment of long-term oxygen therapy (LTOT) criteria.
• Symptoms and signs of right heart failure.
• More than 6 weeks of corticosteroids in the preceding 12 months.
• Combination of other factors e.g. anorexia, greater than 10% weight loss over 6 months, depression, previous NIV/ITU, poor quality of life, increasingly housebound.

In practice in non-malignant disease, a pragmatic and useful way of predicting prognosis is for the senior professional who has known the patient for the longest time to ask him/herself whether or not he/she would be surprised if the patient died within one year.

It appears that the intuitive integration of the many variables that affect prognosis by an experienced clinician is more accurate than scores from prognostic tools.

Table 4.1 BODE Index Score

Body mass index
Obstruction
Dyspnoea
Exercise capacity

	0 point	1 point	2 points	3 points
BMI	>21	≤ 21		
FEV1 % predicted	>65%	50–64%	36–49%	≤ 35%
MRC dyspnoea scale	0–1	2	3	4–5
6-minute walk distance	≥ 350m	250–349m	150–249m	≤ 149m

(Continued)

Table 4.1 (Contd.)

	MRC dyspnoea scale
1	Breathless only with strenuous exercise
2	Short of breath when hurrying on the level or up a slight hill
3	Slower than most people of the same age on a level surface, or
	Have to stop when walking at my own pace on the level
4	Stop for breath walking 100 metres, or
	After walking a few minutes at my own pace on the level
5	Too breathless to leave the house

References

1. Christakis N, Lamond E (2000) Extent and determinants of error in doctors' prognoses in terminally ill patients: prospective cohort study. *Brit Med J*; 320 (7233): 469–472.
2. Celli B, Cote C, Marin J, et al. (2004) The body mass index, airflow obstruction, dyspnoea and exercise capacity index in chronic obstructive pulmonary disease. *N Eng J Med*; 350: 1005–1012.

Recognizing the need for end of life care

'Early recognition of people nearing the end of their life leads to earlier planning and better care.'

Gold Standards Framework, UK

End of life care has been defined on 📖 p. 50. There is no consensus, however, on the definition of the beginning of end of life care. A definition that is too tight may mean that patients requiring end of life care will not receive it. Conversely, lack of a clear definition may be used as an excuse to ignore the fact that a patient may be approaching the end of their life.

Triggers for commencing end of life care

Any of the following scenarios suggest that a patient with incurable disease might need end of life care:

- It would not be surprising if the patient were to die in the next year.
- The patient has developed symptoms that cannot be controlled by disease-modifying treatment.
- The patient needs psychological or spiritual support because of the impact of the disease or limited prognosis.
- The patient has had to make a significant change in social circumstances because of progressive deterioration, such as moving to a care home or sheltered accommodation.
- The patient has had multiple recent admissions to hospital because of deteriorating health.
- The responsible health or social care team judges that the patient requires end of life care.
- The patient requests more intensive care because he/she perceives that the end of life is approaching.
- The patient's carers are experiencing high levels of distress and exhaustion.

A pragmatic approach would be as follows:

- Ask the 'surprise question' ('Would I be surprised if this patient died in the next year?') for all potential patients.
- If the answer is 'no', most patients should be receiving end of life care. The implications of this include the likely need for advance care planning, focusing on enhancing quality of life, basing care in the community, and so on.
- If the answer is 'yes', most patients may not yet be requiring end of life care. However, if a number of the other triggers listed above are true, they are likely to be in need of palliative or supportive care.

The approach described in the definition of end of life care on 📖 p. 50 can simply be viewed as high quality healthcare. The principles it espouses are pertinent to the care of all patients irrespective of diagnosis or prognosis. It is, therefore, never too early to provide this type of care.

Recognition of the terminal phase

The terminal phase is defined as the last few days or hours of a patient's life. A patient in the terminal phase is in the process of dying. The terminal phase can be thought of as the period where even treatment of reversible causes of deterioration cannot change the outcome or its timing.

As the patient gets near to death the following features of dying may be seen:

- Increasing weakness and periods of sleeping, becoming semiconscious.
- Less keen or able to get out of bed.
- Less interested in or aware of things happening around him/her.
- Only able to take sips of fluid; unable to take tablets.
- Sometimes confused, occasionally agitated.

Some of these features will have been present before the terminal phase. Entry into the terminal phase is suggested when most of the above become evident at the same time.

The key challenge of recognizing entry into the terminal phase is that the same clinical features may be seen when a patient has deteriorated from a reversible cause, such as a chest infection. It is vital to do a clinical assessment, taking a history and examining the patient, to exclude reversible causes of decline, before coming to the conclusion that a patient is dying. It may even be necessary to undertake simple investigations. On occasion, a decision may be made not to treat a reversible cause of deterioration. If it is apparent in advance that such a decision will be made, there is clearly no need to search for the underlying cause.

The care of patients in the terminal phase is described in Chapter 12.

Respiratory symptoms

Introduction

Breathlessness, the uncomfortable awareness of the need to breathe, is the most common symptom that troubles dying patients with end-stage respiratory disease. Prevalence is said to reach 90% in patients with advanced lung cancer, and at least 70% in those with COPD and ILD. Clinical management achieves imperfect control and present palliative techniques are certainly less effective than those used in the management of somatic cancer pain.

Nonetheless, there have been significant advances in breathlessness management in the last 10 years, and it is imperative that clinicians who care for patients with respiratory disease at the end of life are familiar with the multi-faceted approach that can improve care. In addition, specialist palliative care services, such as hospices and community teams, are recognizing that they need to provide services to meet the needs of patients with non-malignant disease, of which respiratory disease forms the largest proportion.

Breathlessness is a complex sensation. Physical and psychological components are inextricably linked, so that anxiety and depression at the end of life or associated with the underlying illness can both precipitate and exacerbate episodes of breathlessness. The definition of breathlessness (dyspnoea) most commonly cited is that of the American Thoracic Society (1999):

> Dyspnoea is a term used to characterize a subjective experience of breathing discomfort that consists of qualitatively distinct sensations that vary in intensity. The experience derives from interaction among multiple physiologic, psychological, social, and environmental factors and may induce secondary physiologic and behavioural responses.

The presence of breathlessness is associated with:
- Greater need for sedation to achieve symptom control at the end of life.
- Greater likelihood of hospital admission at this time.
- High levels of distress and exhaustion in family and other informal carers.

Breathlessness is a distressing, frightening sensation and, at the end of life, it is often only possible to reduce its impact, rather than reduce the absolute level of breathlessness.

'Best practice' in the management of breathlessness requires employment of a range of pharmacological and non-pharmacological interventions, tailor-made for the individual, and support for the family and other carers. All this needs to be remembered when planning end of life care; a process that needs to begin once the disease is advanced and progressive, even if this is some months or years before death.

Breathlessness trajectories

Breathlessness tends to follow a different pattern in malignant and non-malignant respiratory disease.

Dyspnoea in malignant disease

Patients with lung cancer (either primary or secondary) or mesothelioma may have felt relatively well until shortly before the diagnosis was made. Having been used to being active, such patients and their families often find the descent into breathlessness on the slightest exertion extremely frightening and disturbing. Their housing and lifestyle will tend not to be already organized to accommodate ill-health.

However, since such patients may have been working or very active until recently, they are less likely to be impoverished, and may have many social contacts able to help them manage the practical difficulties of the illness (such as transport to hospitals, shopping etc.).

Dyspnoea in non-malignant disease

Patients with COPD will typically have been breathless for many years, and many will have had to retire on ill-health grounds. They are likely to have had to withdraw from their social life (through lack of energy but also embarrassment and a sense of stigma). Their spouse or partner will have had to shoulder many extra burdens as well as often losing their own work and financial independence in the process.

As such patients tend to be unable to maintain friendships and social activities (such as churchgoing or being members of clubs or organizations), they often have few friends to help with practical tasks and the end of life phase can lead rapidly to a state of mental and physical exhaustion. Alternatively, such patients and their families may have already moved to a bungalow or started living downstairs or, if living alone, moved to a residential home. All these considerations influence the management of the end of life phase.

Patients with ILD tend to follow the pattern of those with cancer.

Mechanisms of breathlessness

Pathophysiology

Respiration is controlled by a centre within the bulbopontine area of the brainstem, which maintains blood gas and pH values within physiological limits, irrespective of changes in metabolic demand. The respiratory centre receives afferent feedback from a range of chemoreceptors and mechanoreceptors (including lung stretch receptors), which feed into a final common efferent pathway that adjusts respiratory rate and rhythm. Signals from higher centres of the brain (suprapontine areas including the motor cortex and cerebellum) can modify or override these signals. Examples of this include intentional control (e.g. recitation), emotional influences (e.g. anger, fear, laughter), and protective reflexes such as cough.

A schematic model demonstrating the pathophysiology of breathlessness, suitable for use by clinicians, is shown in Figure 5.1. It illustrates that central to an understanding of breathlessness is the recognition that it is a complex sensation influenced, like pain, by the higher centres i.e. thoughts, feelings, and reactions to emotions. This diagram can be a useful aid to explaining breathlessness to patients. It helps demonstrate that psychosocial interventions may be helpful in reducing the impact of breathlessness, even when somatic afferent signals cannot be improved.

If a patient has been living with breathlessness for many years, managing against the odds, and a clinician introduces the concept of psychological interventions, the patient may feel slighted, interpreting the suggestion as implying that he or she is not 'coping'. When psychological interventions are, however, put in the same context as other physical or 'medical' treatments, they may be more easily accepted. It can be explained that a psychological influence, such as fear or anxiety, sends a signal or 'chemical messenger' to the brain, in a similar way to a low oxygen or high carbon dioxide level. Importantly, 'altering central perception' does not imply an inability to 'cope' with the difficulties of breathlessness. It removes the stigma from psychological factors, enabling patients and families to consider dispassionately the possibility of using psychological interventions to help breathlessness.

Perception

The perception of breathlessness as a sensation is still poorly understood. The present consensus is that the brain perceives breathlessness when afferent information reporting the demand for breathing is not matched by afferent information reporting the current level of ventilation. This is called the 'mismatch' theory. The genesis of breathlessness is well reviewed in Booth et al. (2009) and O'Donnell et al. (2007) (see 📖 p. 84).

Breathlessness is composed of qualitatively different sensations, much like pain, but as yet the distinction between these, such as between 'air hunger' and 'work of breathing', have not been found to be useful in defining aetiology. There is, however, a growing understanding that 'air hunger' is more distressing than increased work of breathing.

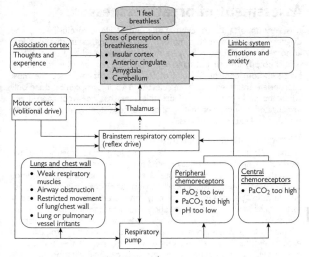

Fig. 5.1 Pathophysiology of breathlessness[1].

Reference

1. Moosavi S. Pathophysiology of breathlessness. In: Cambridge Breathlessness Intervention Service Manual. Cambridge University Hospitals NHS Foundation Trust. http://www.cuh.org.uk/btreathlessness

Assessment of breathlessness

It is very important that, even at the end of life, a careful history and diagnosis is made of each symptom. This does not mean that a patient at home, hospital, or in a hospice should be subjected to a spiral CT or bronchoscopy in their last days. It is, however, only possible to give the best symptom control and end of life care to patients once the most appropriate treatment has been selected. This, in turn, can be done only when the underlying cause of breathlessness has been considered and investigated, in a manner that is, of course, consistent with an individual's situation and expressed wishes.

Change in pattern of breathlessness

A change in pattern of the symptom must lead to reassessment of the working diagnosis. New onset or rapid progression of breathlessness may mean that a reversible cause of breathlessness has developed, in addition to the intractable disease. Specialist investigation may give the best 'risk benefit ratio' (perhaps more accurately considered as 'short-term discomfort versus longer-term comfort ratio'), even near the end of life.

In situations where further investigation is inappropriate, a good history, coupled where necessary with specialist advice on the probability of each differential diagnosis, is likely to give that patient the best chance of effective symptom control. In contrast, a 'catch-all' diagnosis of 'dying from respiratory disease' combined with the prescription of 'broad brush' pharmacological treatment will never be in a patient's best interests.

Discussion of treatment options

It is vital to discuss the options for the diagnosis and treatment of potential complications with patients, to determine their preferences and to record and communicate these widely (letters to GP, Preferred Priorities of Care document etc.). This level of communication should be instigated early and then maintained (see 📖 Chapter 8 pp. 174–176). This will make it much more likely that a patient with a life-threatening illness is given the type of care they would prefer, rather than interventions chosen as a reaction to a given clinical state, resulting, for example, in unwanted invasive treatment such as ventilation.

Collaboration with colleagues

Keeping in contact with other clinicians caring for a dying patient is essential, and written letters are usually too slow when the active dying phase has started. Keep in touch with colleagues directly in 'real time' using telephone, email, or fax, so that the patient and family do not get conflicting messages from different clinicians. Frequent contact between specialist and primary care services is integral to the provision of high quality care.

- Respiratory specialists and general practitioners (GPs) may be fortunate enough to have a relationship with their patients over many years. This is usually tremendously valuable as the end of life approaches. It may, however, occasionally be hazardous as symptoms can be automatically ascribed to previously experienced conditions, rather than reconsidered anew.

- It is important that non-respiratory specialists, for example in palliative medicine or general practice, do not neglect to seek advice from respiratory physicians. The converse is also true.
- Telephone consultations can be of great value, for example when a very ill patient at home or in a hospice is unable to attend a hospital outpatient appointment.

Assessment tool

Although there is, as yet, no perfect assessment tool for breathlessness, the recently developed Dyspnoea-12 shows great promise. It is short and therefore not burdensome for breathless patients with limited ability to concentrate, and has been carefully designed using modern understanding of questionnaire development. It has been widely validated in patients with non-malignant disease, and further work is currently being undertaken in patients with cancer.[1]

Table 5.1 Dyspnoea-12 questionnaire

This questionnaire is designed to help us learn more about how your breathing is troubling you. Please read each item and then tick in the box that best matches your breathing **these days.** If you do not experience an item tick the 'none' box. Please respond to all items. (Score 0–3 for each item, maximum score 36)

Item	None	Mild	Moderate	Severe
1. My breath does not go in all the way				
2. My breathing requires more work				
3. I feel short of breath				
4. I have difficulty catching my breath				
5. I cannot get enough air				
6. My breathing is uncomfortable				
7. My breathing is exhausting				
8. My breathing makes me feel depressed				
9. My breathing makes me feel miserable				
10. My breathing is distressing				
11. My breathing makes me agitated				
12. My breathing is irritating				

Reference

1. Yorke J, Moosavi SH, Shuldham C, Jones PW (2010) Quantification of dyspnoea using descriptors: development and initial testing of the Dyspnoea-12. *Thorax*; 65: 21–26.

Principles of management of breathlessness

The multidimensional pathophysiology of dyspnoea gives scope to a wide range of potential approaches to palliate the symptom. Interventions act in a number of ways, including reversing the underlying cause, reducing ventilatory demand, optimizing the mechanics of ventilation, and modifying the central perception of breathlessness.

Principles of symptom management are outlined first below, followed by more detail on non-pharmacological and pharmacological approaches.

Reversal of underlying cause(s)

This is not always possible in patients with advanced and incurable disease. However, potentially reversible conditions causing or exacerbating the symptom should always be considered and, if appropriate, searched for. Common examples of reversible causes of deteriorating breathlessness in such patients include:

• infection
• anaemia
• pulmonary embolism
• pleural effusion.

A degree of anxiety is inevitably present in patients suffering from breathlessness. Eliciting and addressing patients' concerns and fears compassionately can be very effective as an initial management strategy. Patients (and their carers) may have seen many different clinicians over the years, and never yet had the chance to 'tell the full story' of the impact of breathlessness on their lives. Even for patients to understand that, although feeling breathless is extremely unpleasant, it does not actually harm the patient, can be extremely helpful; it is this fear that causes patients to remain inactive to avoid provoking breathlessness, therefore becoming deconditioned.

Non-pharmacological approaches

These tend to be the most useful interventions in breathless patients with advanced but not end-stage disease. The techniques are safe, can be very effective, and give patients a sense of control of their symptom. However, any non-pharmacological approach needs regular practice to be effective and to remain so, and patients in the last weeks and days of life usually lack the energy or time to do this. The success of these interventions depends largely on the extent to which a patient engages with them. (See 📖 pp. 68–74.)

Pharmacological approaches

Drugs such as opioids and benzodiazepines have an important role in palliating breathlessness in patients with advanced disease and at the end of life, who may benefit less from non-drug measures (see 📖 pp. 78–80).

Oxygen tends to be overused in this patient group. A small proportion of patients may gain relief of breathlessness. An individual clinical assessment is often necessary, as there are no reliable criteria to help predict which patients may benefit (see pp. 76–77). Most patients, however, regardless of whether or not they are hypoxaemic, will gain benefit from using a fan (see p. 69).

Table 5.2 Management of chronic intractable breathlessness

Non-pharmacological treatments: suitable for all breathless patients	• Facial cooling with a hand-held fan (aim at area subserved by Vth cranial nerve around mouth, nose and surrounding cheeks) • Keeping physically active, exercise programmes for suitable patients, tailored to that person • Breathing re-training • Relaxation and anxiety control techniques • Psychological support for patient and carer (very frightening to watch someone being breathless) • Addressing fears about breathlessness • Education about the symptom
Pharmacological treatment: more important in the severely breathless	Palliative treatment: oral opioids reduce breathlessness by about 20% in many patients, start low and increase slowly to reduce incidence of adverse effects. More useful in patients with severe breathlessness. • Opioid naïve patients: slow titration phase starting as low as 1mg daily, increasing 1mg daily each week until on 5-10mg morphine sulphate MR bd and using 2.5mg prn. • Already taking opioids: increase current dose by 25% and encourage use of prn opioids for breathlessness. Oral benzodiazepines (e.g. lorazepam) or phenothiazines may be helpful if patients cannot use non-pharmacological anxiety-reducing strategies. At the end of life: prescribe continuous subcutaneous infusion of morphine/diamorphine and midazolam. • Opioid naïve patients: typical regimen would be 2.5-5.0 mg diamorphine with 5–10mg midazolam over 24 hours. • Already taking opioids: add midazolam (5–10mg) or levomepromazine (6.25–12.5 mg, more if anxiety very prominent). **Oxygen** In patients with advanced disease and chronic intractable breathlessness, there is no evidence that oxygen is better than a fan, unless the patient desaturates below 90% on exercise.

Non-pharmacological interventions

Non-pharmacological interventions are of particular value in the management of breathlessness when patients are mobile. They need to be learned early and practised regularly in order to be useful.

Both non-pharmacological and pharmacological interventions have their place in the treatment of breathlessness. When a patient is first diagnosed with advanced respiratory disease a range of non-pharmacological interventions should be instituted. These can include exercise, a fan, anxiety reduction techniques, and other psychological interventions. Encouraging mental and social activity, although not widely recognized as a health intervention, can have a positive impact on well-being. As the patient becomes less well, pharmacological therapy is likely to be needed.

Pulmonary rehabilitation

Pulmonary rehabilitation is an important intervention in the management of breathlessness in advanced respiratory disease. There is strong evidence that it improves breathlessness, as well as fatigue, anxiety, and quality of life. All breathless patients should be offered an assessment.

It is important to understand that pulmonary rehabilitation is not an intervention just for patients with a longer prognosis. There is evidence that rehabilitation can benefit patients with the most advanced disease, including those that are too breathless to leave the house (MRC dyspnoea score 5), and even patients that are dependent on invasive ventilation.[1,2] In addition, there is gathering evidence that short, low-intensity, and home-based programmes can lead to benefit.[3]

Some patients will need support or encouragement to accept pulmonary rehabilitation and sometimes a home visit or attendance at a hospice breathlessness clinic will give patients the confidence to participate.

Exercise outside pulmonary rehabilitation

Exercise is one of the most effective non-pharmacological interventions for breathlessness and is based on the greatest evidence base. Although patients with far advanced disease may be too unwell to join a formal exercise or rehabilitation programme, it is still vital to encourage activity. Simple activity such as getting up out of a chair and walking to the television in the 'advert breaks' (for example) has many benefits, including:
- maintenance of independence
- reduction of burden on carers
- increased confidence and self-efficacy
- reduction in the 'humiliation' (which many feel) of being dependent on others
- generation of a rare sense of progress or improvement.

It is particularly important in patients with advanced progressive disease that exercise is not viewed as compulsory, with the insinuation that it may improve prognosis. Exercise may, therefore, be best described as 'activity'.

Psychosocial activity, such as attending a hospice day centre, may be just as important.

Patients may have withdrawn from social life partly because they feel stigmatized by breathlessness, coughing, or their oxygen equipment, or because it drains too much energy. Once they understand that activity may do more good than harm, they may feel more able to re-engage with the outside world, relieving to some extent the tedium of chronic ill-health and reducing stress in the home.

Encourage patients to consider exercise and social activity as health-promoting strategies that can improve quality of life.

Passive exercise

Transcutaneous neuromuscular electrical stimulation (NMES) leads to passive exercise by electrical stimulation of muscle groups, such as the quadriceps. There is consistent evidence in patients with COPD that it can increase muscle strength and exercise capacity, and reduce dyspnoea during activities of daily living.[4] Research evaluating the role of NMES in palliation of breathlessness in advanced cancer is currently being undertaken.

Although not yet in widespread use, NMES has the potential to be a useful intervention in patients with far advanced disease:

- Treatment is home-based and feasible for patients who are chair-bound by severe breathlessness.
- The intervention is very well tolerated.
- Physiotherapists are generally trained in the use of NMES.
- Equipment is relatively inexpensive.

'NMES is an exciting intervention ripe for adaptation to the palliative-care setting.'

Sachs (2009)[3]

The handheld fan

- This simple, cheap, and portable piece of equipment is an immensely valuable tool in reducing breathlessness and improving self-efficacy.
- Its use is supported by evidence from healthy volunteer studies, and emerging evidence in cardiopulmonary disease.[5]
- It is thought that the cooling of nasal receptors and parts of the face innervated by the 2nd and 3rd branches of the trigeminal cranial nerve transmits a signal to the brainstem respiratory complex, which alters the central perception of breathlessness.
- The handheld fan is usually much preferred by patients to bedside fans, which can cause discomfort from excessive draught.
- It is easy to use even for patients with end-stage disease and, unlike oxygen, does not stigmatize its user or have any known adverse effects.
- Handheld fans with three or more rotating blades seem to be most effective.

It is important never simply to hand the fan to patients without explanation as they will tend not to believe that such an 'everyday object' could be helpful. Its use should always be demonstrated, and the following points can be made to enhance the psychological impact of its use.

Instructions for use of handheld fan
- Use it whenever you feel yourself becoming breathless.
- Try to adopt a comfortable position, such as sitting leaning forward slightly, and hold the fan approximately 30cm (12in) from your face.
- Aim the draught of air towards the central part of your face so that you feel it around the sides of your nose and above your top lip.
- You should feel the benefit within a few minutes.
- It will not alter the disease or the cause of breathlessness, but will shorten attacks of breathlessness.
- There is scientific evidence to support its use.
- Try to take a fan with you when you are out, and also have one in different parts of your house, so that you do not have to search for one when breathless.
- By having a way of reducing breathlessness and regaining a degree of control, you are no longer simply waiting helplessly for another breathlessness attack. This is helpful in itself.

A video demonstrating the use of the handheld fan and a patient information sheet can be accessed at http://www.cuh.org.uk/breathlessness.

Breathing exercises
- A specialist physiotherapist can analyse and suggest changes to patients' respiratory patterns, and recommend more comfortable positions for breathing and for recovering from episodes of breathlessness.
- All clinicians helping breathless patients need to be able to demonstrate abdominal breathing, although a physiotherapist or occupational therapist may do this more skilfully than others.
- Techniques need to be practised to have maximum impact. Practice during pulmonary rehabilitation or hospice day therapy can be helpful.

Instructions to reduce respiratory rate and prolong expiration
- Position yourself comfortably. Relax your body and mind.
- Inhale deeply and smoothly for four units of time. Fill your lungs completely, and feel your abdomen distend.
- Hold your breath for a count of two units of time and then exhale for a count of seven.
- Concentrate on a smooth (not 'snatched') in-breath, and a long and relaxed out-breath. Focus on the out breath.

Some patients find visualization helpful. Consider visualizing blowing into a balloon, the balloon steadily expanding on breathing out, and sucking in on breathing in. Alternatively, imagine breathing in 'good things' and breathing out the 'bad or harmful things' from the body.

Instructions for diaphragmatic breathing
- Sit in your most comfortable position, and put one hand on your chest and one on your stomach.
- Slowly inhale through your nose or through pursed lips. As you inhale, feel your stomach expand with your hand.
- Slowly exhale through pursed lips to regulate the release of air.
- Rest and repeat.

There are other breathing techniques that may be useful, including positions to adopt that improve the mechanical efficiency of breathlessness (such as sitting up, leaning forward slightly). Patients must have an individual assessment from an experienced respiratory physiotherapist to gain maximum benefit. Further information is available on the Breathlessness Intervention Service website (http://www.cuh.org.uk/breathlessness) and in the associated Breathlessness Manual.[6]

Energy conservation

Many breathless patients continue to expect to achieve as much as they could before they were ill and at the same rate. Many will admit to feeling impatient, frustrated, and angry at the restrictions imposed by the illness and express disbelief at the degree to which their daily activities are limited.

Occupational therapists are particularly helpful in helping patients pace their activities and conserve energy for more enjoyable pursuits. They may also be able to recommend useful equipment. Walking aids, for example, have been shown to reduce the impact of breathlessness[4]

The following advice and guidance can be helpful for patients:
- It is necessary to accept the reality of the illness ('Yes, this is happening. Yes, people can sometimes feel breathless merely on dressing.').
- Adopting a slower pace can sometimes allow one to achieve more.
- Try to rest between periods of activity.
- Spread out activities over a week rather than over a day.
- It is important to try to continue being active, even in the face of discouragement.
- It may be necessary to ask for help or support, such as using a wheelchair at social events or hiring a hotel room rather than travelling to an event on the day.
- Early and detailed planning of ambitious social outings can be very helpful.
- Energy can be considered to be contained in an energy tank rather like a petrol tank; it is helpful to be reminded not to run 'on empty'.

Anxiety reduction

Anxiety increases breathlessness, which in turn contributes to the anxiety, leading to a deteriorating vicious cycle. Anxiety associated with chronic intractable breathlessness appears to be even more common than depression, and possibly more long lasting.

Anxiety reduction techniques are a skill that can help with many of the vicissitudes of chronic, advancing illness. However, learning them is time-consuming and requires commitment. They should be taught and practised as early as possible in the course of respiratory disease, as learning new techniques becomes increasingly difficult with advancing ill-health. The technique should be chosen for and tailored to the individual patient. This may take some trial and error. The range of techniques includes:

- progressive muscular relaxation
- visualization or guided imagery
- cognitive behavioural therapy (CBT)
- self-hypnosis
- mindfulness
- breathing pattern recognition and modification
- distraction e.g. by music
- yoga.

Some techniques are particularly useful at the time of a breathless attack (e.g. visualization, CBT), and others are of value in reducing background levels of stress and anxiety (e.g. yoga, mindfulness). A practical approach to some of these techniques is contained in the box on 📖 p. 73.

Ritual for crises

One of the most important aspects of caring for a breathless patient is to listen to exactly what the patient is experiencing when breathless. Talking through typical episodes from inception to resolution can reveal unhelpful thoughts or ideas that may be exacerbating the anxiety associated with breathlessness. Carers should be involved in this process as it is natural to feel particularly helpless and frightened watching a family member suffering with breathlessness. Some report literally 'not knowing what to do' when their loved one becomes breathless.

Designing a 'ritual for crises' may help to avert out of hours hospital admission. It may encompass such very simple ideas as 'When you become breathless, sit down. Your wife can give you the fan and switch it on, and you may find it helpful if she puts her hand on your arm.'

Patients and carers should be taught how to detect exacerbations early. Reinforcing or 'role playing' these scenarios can help prevent a crisis developing.

See 📖 Chapter 6 p. 119 for a cognitive behavioural therapy approach to controlling panic and breathlessness.

Non-invasive ventilation

NIV is most commonly used to increase survival and palliate symptoms in patients with acute, potentially reversible respiratory failure (e.g. infective exacerbation of COPD) and in those with respiratory failure due to neuromuscular or chest wall conditions.

It is, however, increasingly being recognized as a potential method for palliating breathlessness, particularly in patients with intolerable adverse effects from drugs such as opioids.[7] Use of NIV is described in more detail in 📖 Chapter 2 pp. 40–42, including its role in 'buying time' at the very end of life, when a patient wishes to achieve a specific goal.

Progressive muscular relaxation

- The patient actively tenses and relaxes specific parts of the body in a progressive order.
- Start with tensing and relaxing the whole body, and then move progressively through the body, for example, jaw (clench), tongue (stick out), shoulders (hunched), hands (fists) etc.
- It is helpful if the clinician guides the patient through the exercise, pacing and modelling the technique.
- 'I wonder if you can lift up your shoulders, lift them up to your ears, hold them there, squeeze them tightly, and then let them drop down, just let them flop… then once more hunch them up, hold it… then let them go, feel all the tight tension in your shoulders just drain away… Now, clench your hands into fists…' and so on.

Visualization

- One form of imagery is for a patient, relaxed and with their eyes shut, to be guided to think of a place or an activity where he or she has felt safe and happy in the past.
- The patient is encouraged to recall the details of the scene, using all five senses: sight, sound, smell, feel, and taste.
- The clinician may choose to elaborate on the description of the patient, contributing to the experience of distraction and relaxation.
- 'You can feel the granules of sand under your feet as you step steadily along the beach… the ripples of water sooth your feet and sound musical and you can feel the sun making your skin warm… the smell of clean sea air is refreshing you… you feel free…' and so on.

Principles of cognitive behavioural therapy

- Formal CBT can only be provided by a qualified practitioner. However, all professionals can encourage patients to describe their thoughts, feelings, behaviours, and physical symptoms and explore how they may be linked.
- Revealing a vicious cycle can be a powerful way of explaining problems to patients, for example, how fear of dying can lead to anxiety, which worsens breathlessness, making the fear of dying even greater.
- Writing down pertinent thoughts, feelings etc. and using arrows to graphically demonstrate the links can be helpful, both through acknowledging their existence and showing their interrelationships.

Mindfulness and mindful breathing

- Mindfulness is derived from the Buddhist practice of meditation. With practice, individuals learn to develop a non-judging awareness and acceptance of the present moment. It can reduce rumination on the past and anxiety about the future.
- Mindful breathing focuses on the present physical sensation of breathing, helping patients to live with and accept their experience of breathing, rather than fearing or avoiding thinking about it.
- Following a CD describing mindful techniques can be very helpful for patients.

References

1. Evans R, Singh S, Collier R, Williams JE, Morgan MD (2009) Pulmonary rehabilitation is successful for COPD irrespective of MRC dyspnoea grade. *Respir Med*; 103 (7): 1070–1075.
2. Martin U, Hincapie L, Nimchuk M et al. (2005) Impact of whole-body rehabilitation in patients receiving chronic mechanical ventilation. *Crit Care Med*; 33 (10): 2259–2265.
3. Sachs S, Weinberg R (2009) Pulmonary rehabilitation for dyspnoea in the palliative care setting. *Curr Opinion Supp Pall Care*; 3: 112–119.
4. Bausewein C, Booth S, Gysels M, Higginson I. Non-pharmacological interventions for breathlessness in advanced stages of malignant and non-malignant disease. Cochrane Database SystRev 2008 Issue 2 CD 005623.
5. Galbraith S, Fagan P, Perkins P, Lynch A, Booth S (2010) Does the use of a handheld fan improve chronic dypsnoea? A randomized controlled cross-over trial. *J Pain Sy Manage*; 39: 831–838.
6. Booth S, Burkin J, Moffat C (2010) Cambridge Breathlessness Intervention Service Manual. Cambridge University Hospitals NHS Foundation Trust http:// www.cuh.org.uk/breathlessness
7. Shee C, Green M (2003) Non invasive ventilation and palliation: experience in a district general hospital and a review. *Palliat Med*; 17: 21–26.

Oxygen therapy

Long-term oxygen therapy (LTOT)

Use of continuous oxygen for 15 or more hours each 24 hours is well established in severely hypoxic patients with COPD (see 🕮 Chapter 2 pp. 38–39). Although LTOT is used primarily because of its benefit on survival, there is also evidence that it improves quality of life and reduces severity of breathlessness.

The prescription of oxygen concentrators for long-term use is now undertaken by specialist respiratory clinics in the UK and follows strict guidelines.

Short-burst oxygen therapy (SBOT)

SBOT is arguably the most overused intervention for palliating breathlessness. There is an increasing body of evidence from controlled trials that it is not significantly more effective than a flow of air. Furthermore, limiting use of oxygen to only those patients that gain benefit could lead to massive financial savings.

The role of oxygen in the palliation of breathlessness is still controversial in both malignant and non-malignant disease. Current controlled trial evidence suggests the following:
- A draught of cool air is helpful in reducing breathlessness.
- Oxygen tends to be no more effective than a flow of cool air, irrespective of a patient's initial level of hypoxaemia or nonmoxaemia.
- A few patients may benefit from SBOT, particularly when used during exertion (ambulatory oxygen).
- There is no way of predicting, without an individual clinical assessment, which patients will gain benefit.

It is now standard specialist palliative care practice to offer a fan first (see 🕮 p. 69). Oxygen is only prescribed when there are other indicators, such as significant desaturation on exercise. An individual clinical assessment is always necessary to determine which patients will benefit from oxygen.

The burdens of oxygen therapy are considerable:
- A degree of psychological dependence is inevitable, and some patients become acutely anxious during even a short interruption in oxygen supply.
- Cumbersome and heavy equipment can restrict movement, activities within the home, and excursions outside the home.
- An oxygen mask can impair communication between a patient and their family.
- Some patients feel a sense of social stigma and embarrassment, further compounding social isolation.
- It is both expensive and highly combustible.

Very ill or dying patients may resume smoking or, indeed, may never have never given up. Relatives and friends often smoke. Oxygen is extremely hazardous in smoking households, and patients and family may need to be repeatedly warned about this. It may be safer to remove oxygen under these circumstances.

Heliox

There is some evidence that Heliox 28 (72% helium and 28% oxygen) may help reduce dyspnoea and increase oxygenation in conditions where there is increased work of breathing, such as with COPD or asthma.

One small feasibility trial compared Heliox with oxygen-enriched air in 12 patients with lung cancer, and showed an improvement in breathlessness on exertion and exercise tolerance.[1] However, stronger evidence is needed before Heliox can be recommended as standard treatment for the palliation of breathlessness. Furthermore, the logistical challenges of administration, including access to gas and equipment as well as significant costs, would make routine use in end of life care difficult.

Reference

1. Ahmedzai S, Laude E, Robertson A, Troy G, Vora V (2004) A double-blind, randomised, controlled phase II trial of Heliox 28 gas mixture in lung cancer patients with dyspnoea on exertion. *Br J Cancer;* 90: 366–371.

Pharmacological management

Opioids

Although once feared as a cause of respiratory depression, oral morphine is the mainstay of pharmacological treatment for intractable breathlessness. Its use is supported by the greatest weight of evidence and extensive clinical experience.

- Opioids seem to give approximately a 20% improvement in breathlessness from baseline in those whom they help.
- They seem to work best in the most severely breathless patients.
- There is still uncertainty in a number of areas including the most effective opioid, route, and formulation (e.g. immediate or modified release).
- Oral morphine is the opioid most widely used for breathlessness. Fentanyl may have a role because of its rapid onset of action (for example, sublingual or intranasal). However, its use is not recommended without specialist advice and probably inpatient observation, in those unused to prescribing it.

Commencing opioids in breathless patients

For opioid naïve patients in the community, opioids should be commenced at a very low dose, morphine sulphate immediate release (IR) 0.5–1.5mg bd, with the same dose as required as a 'top up'. This can be increased each week by 1mg per day, until a daily dose of 10mg has been reached. At this point the patient can be converted to morphine sulphate modified release (MR) 5mg bd.

The use of low doses and slow titration makes this regimen suitable for patients with COPD. Patients with interstitial lung disease (ILD) may particularly benefit from opioids, as they often have stimulation of their respiratory centres (with hypoxaemia but rarely hypercapnia). Again, opioids can be commenced in the community using this regimen.

Patients already on opioids (for example with cancer and pain) can use the same 'as required' dose for breathlessness as they do for pain. The regular opioid dose may need to increase. The choice of timing of 'as required' doses can give patients a sense of control and self-efficacy, and contribute to the benefit experienced.

All patients should be reassessed at weekly intervals, in person or by telephone. Simple quantitative measures of effectiveness can be used even during telephone consultations, for example, a numerical rating scale (NRS) with anchors such as 'no breathlessness' and 'breathlessness as bad as can be', or a BORG scale of 'average breathlessness over last week'.

High-risk patients, such as those with previous episodes of CO_2 retention during exacerbations or with type II respiratory failure, should generally be admitted to the local hospice or respiratory unit for observation, allowing a more rapid titration period.

Concerns about opioids

The adverse effects of opioids are considered in detail in 📖 Chapter 6 pp. 102–107. The following points are, however, worth noting:

- Patients should be warned about adverse effects. Nausea tends to settle in a few days and can be treated with anti-emetics. All patients

on opioids should be commenced on laxatives, and the dose titrated to the degree of constipation experienced.
- Patients with non-malignant disease may fear that prescription of opioids implies the presence of cancer. Both patients and relatives may need specific reassurance.
- Clinicians tend to be concerned about the possibility of respiratory depression. There has been no evidence to date that clinically significant respiratory depression does occur, and oral opioids started at a low dose and slowly titrated are very safe. Patients can be alerted to the potential risk and advised that respiratory depression would be preceded by sedation (with slow titration), providing a 'built-in' safety mechanism. Patients should be told not to take the next opioid dose if excessively sleepy, and to seek medical advice. Written information for patients and close communication with the community team can both be very helpful.

Benzodiazepines

Benzodiazepines (BDZ) are regularly prescribed in breathless patients with advanced disease. The theoretical basis for their use is clear; they are anxiolytic drugs, and anxiety can precipitate or exacerbate breathlessness. However, there is little research evidence to support their use, and rigorous controlled trials are urgently needed.[1]

BDZ are rarely used in patients with non-malignant disease and a potentially long prognosis because of their potential to create dependency. Non-pharmacological interventions for breathlessness are generally favoured. However, patients with cancer frequently use BDZ, as the risk of dependency is of less concern.

Lorazepam (sublingual) and midazolam (subcutaneous) are the BDZ most commonly used in this context. Diazepam can also be used, but it has a particularly long half-life with active metabolites that persist for even longer, which can lead to accumulation and prolonged sedation. Please see 📖 Chapter 6 p. 118 for further details of these drugs.

Buspirone

There is a small amount of evidence that buspirone may reduce anxiety and breathlessness in patients with COPD. However, its usefulness is limited by the fact that it takes 2–4 weeks to work. See 📖 Chapter 6 p. 118 for further details.

Phenothiazines

Whereas in the UK BDZ tend to be used to supplement opioids, in Canada and the USA the phenothiazine, levomepromazine, is more commonly used for the pharmacological treatment of anxiety. Levomepromazine has a broad spectrum of receptor activity, which leads to a range of benefits (including anti-emetic effect) as well as adverse effects (including sedation, dysphoria, and hypotension). There is little published evidence to support the use of phenothiazines in breathlessness. The major tranquillizer effect suggests that it would be most useful in patients experiencing real terror associated with breathlessness.

Antidepressants

Depression is prevalent in advanced respiratory disease, and is frequently under-diagnosed (see 📖 Chapter 6 pp. 120–121). It is well recognized that mood states and emotional factors influence the central perception of breathlessness, and there are some data to suggest that there are serotonergic pathways in the brainstem respiratory centre.

Although there is very limited evidence for the efficacy of antidepressants in breathlessness, the use of anti-depressants to improve low mood may be helpful for breathlessness because of the significant impact of mood on symptom perception.

- On initial assessment, all breathless patients should be screened for depression (see 📖 Chapter 6 pp. 120–121).
- Antidepressants tend to take at least 2 weeks to develop a therapeutic effect. They would be of very little value in escalating breathlessness near the very end of life.
- Selective serotonin reuptake inhibitors are the most commonly used first-line anti-depressant e.g. citalopram 10–20mg od. Fluoxetine should be avoided as it may increase anxiety.
- Mirtazapine, a centrally active presynaptic α2 adrenergic receptor antagonist, is being increasingly used in patients with advanced disease. As well as its antidepressant effect, it has a range of benefits including reduction in anxiety, improvement of sleep, and treatment of neuropathic pain. Start with a dose of 15mg at night (this dose has an anxiolytic effect equivalent to 15mg diazepam).

Inhaled furosemide

Several small studies have investigated the possible effectiveness of inhaled furosemide in dyspnoea after anecdotal reports of remarkable relief in some patients. There is not enough evidence to recommend its use outside clinical trials or specialist centres at present.

Reference

1. Simon S, Bausewein C, Booth S, Harding R, Higginson IJ (2008) Benzodiazepines for the relief of breathlessness in malignant and advanced non-malignant diseases in adults (Protocol). *The Cochrane Library*, Issue 4.

Cough

Intractable cough is a challenging symptom that is not easily treated. It can cause many problems including sleep disturbance, embarrassment, precipitation of episodes of breathlessness, muscle strain, rib fractures, urinary incontinence, vomiting, and retinal haemorrhage. It has a significantly negative impact on quality of life.

Chronic cough is highly prevalent in patients with advanced respiratory disease, and rates of up to 80% have been reported, both in patients with COPD and in those with lung cancer.

Aetiology

In COPD, there is evidence that cough is triggered by airway inflammation. Some inflammatory mediators, such as prostaglandins, are known to be tussive agents. Mucus hypersecretion and impaired ciliary clearance also contribute, particularly in smokers. Smoking cessation reduces the prevalence of cough in patients with COPD significantly.

Malignant lung disease may trigger cough through airway infiltration, distortion, or obstruction.

Co-morbidities frequently contribute to cough:
• Post-nasal drip.
• Chest infection/bronchiectasis.
• Gastro-oesophageal reflux.
• Cardiac failure.
• Vocal cord paralysis (malignant recurrent laryngeal nerve involvement).

Medical intervention can also cause cough, in particular ACE inhibitors, β-blockers, methotrexate, and radiotherapy-induced pneumonitis or fibrosis.

Assessment

The following key questions must be answered:
• What is causing the cough?
• Are any of the potential causes reversible?
• Is the cough 'wet' or 'dry'?

Management

Correct reversible causes

This is the most effective treatment of cough. Treatment of underlying infection is vital. Sub-clinical gastro-oesophageal reflux disease (GORD) is common. Simple anti-reflux measures, such as wearing loose clothing and avoiding precipitating foods, and a trial of acid suppression (e.g. proton pump inhibitor therapy) should be considered.

Simple remedies

Keeping the throat moist and coated with sugar (for example with sweets or hot sugary drinks) may reduce the hyper-reflexivity of the cough reflex. Simple linctus (e.g. 5mL tds), a soothing demulcent, can also be used. Although there is sparse research evidence to support their use, these simple interventions do appear to help.

Wet cough

Expectoration of sputum should be encouraged in patients with a wet cough. Physiotherapy, nebulized saline, or steam inhalation can all be helpful. Patients can be taught to 'huff', forcing expiration from a low–medium lung volume, to help clear secretions. A mucolytic drug that can reduce the viscosity of secretions, such as carbocysteine 750mg tds, can benefit some patients.

The only time a wet cough should be suppressed is in an imminently dying patient, where the cough is too weak to expectorate sputum (see below).

Dry cough

A dry cough serves no physiological purpose and can be suppressed. Opioids can provide centrally acting cough suppression and appear to be the most effective intervention. Use can be limited by adverse effects, and opioids may be of particular value in breathless patients who would anyway benefit from opioids. Examples of drugs and doses include:

- codeine linctus 15mg (5mL) tds to qds
- morphine sulphate IR solution 2.5mg qds and prn.

There is evidence of some benefit from inhaled sodium cromoglicate from one small trial in patients with lung cancer. Further definitive studies are needed.

- Sodium cromoglicate 10mg qds (inhaled via spacer).

Further reading

Abernethy AP, McDonald CF, Frith PA et al Effect of palliative oxygen versus room air in relief of breathlessness in patients with refractory dyspnoea: a double-blind randomised controlled trial. *The Lancet* 2001; 376 (9743): 784–793.

American Thoracic Society (1999) Dyspnea. Mechanisms, assessment and management: a consensus statement. *Am J Respir Crit Care Med* 159: 321–340.

Booth S, Bausewein C, Higginson IJ, Moosavi S (2009) The pharmacological treatment of refractory breathlessness. *Expert Rev Respir Med*; 3: 21–36.

Bausewein C, Booth S, Higginson IJ (2008) Measurement of dyspnoea in the clinical rather than the research setting. *Current Opinion in Supportive and Palliative Care*; 2: 95–99.

Booth S, Moosavi SH, Higginson IJ (2008) The aetiology and management of intractable breathlessness in patients with advanced cancer: with a systematic review of pharmacological and inhaled therapy. *Nature Clinical Practice Oncology*; 5 (2): 90–100.

Breitbart W, Payne D, Passik S (2005) Psychological and psychiatric interventions in pain control. In: Doyle D, Hanks G, Cherny N, Calman K (eds.), *Oxford Textbook of Palliative Medicine*, 3rd edition. Oxford University Press, Oxford, pp424–438.

Hosnieh F, Morice AH (2008) Cough in palliative care. *Progress in Palliative Care* 16 (1): 31–37.

Jennings AL, Davies AN, Higgins JP, Gibbs JS, Broadley KE. (2002) A systematic review of the use of opioids in the management of dyspnoea. *Thorax* 57: 939–944.

O'Donnell DE, Banzett RB, Carrieri-Kohlman V, et al. (2007) Pathophysiology of dyspnea in chronic obstructive pulmonary disease: a Roundtable. *Am Thoracic Society*; 4: 145–168.

Segal Z, Williams J, Teasdale J (2002) *Mindfulness-based Cognitive Therapy for Depression*. The Guildford Press, New York.

Smith J, Woodcock A (2006) Cough and its importance in COPD. *International Journal of COPD*; 1 (3): 305–314.

Spathis A, Booth S (2008) End of life care in chronic obstructive pulmonary disease: in search of a good death. *International Journal of COPD*; 3 (1): 1–19.

Chapter 6

Non-respiratory symptoms

Introduction

Breathlessness is the most prevalent symptom experienced by patients with advanced respiratory disease. It is an expected consequence of chest pathology, and clinicians understandably tend to focus on controlling this symptom above all others.

It is imperative, however, that attention is also given to non-respiratory symptoms. Fatigue, insomnia, pain, anorexia, anxiety, and depression are each experienced by the majority of patients in the last year of life. Such symptoms contribute significantly to patients' poor quality of life.

The greatest priority of patients approaching the end of life and their carers is to avoid dying in distress with uncontrolled symptoms.

Symptom burden

The symptom burden experienced by those with advanced respiratory disease is considerable. Whereas it is well established that patients with advanced lung cancer tend to experience a range of non-respiratory symptoms, clinicians fail to appreciate that those with benign disease suffer a remarkably similar symptom burden.[1]

- In both chronic respiratory disease (CRD) and lung cancer (LC), the mean number of symptoms per patient is seven.
- The mean number of 'very distressing' symptoms is two in both groups.

Table 3.1 (see 📖 p. 45) documents the prevalence of symptoms in both patients with benign and patients with malignant advanced respiratory disease.

- Those with CRD suffer more breathlessness, anxiety, and depression.
- Patients with LC develop more pain, anorexia, and constipation.

Principles of symptom control

These principles apply to the management of all symptoms.

- Aim to find the underlying cause and treat any reversible causes.
- Be proactive, ask direct questions, and do not wait for the patient to complain.
- Treat promptly, as neglected symptoms deteriorate and become harder to manage.
- Reassess repeatedly until symptom free.
- Make one change at a time if possible, so that it is easier to establish which change has been useful.

The principles that underpin palliative care are also of value.

- Consider the contribution of psychosocial and spiritual factors. For example, addressing a mistaken belief that the symptom reflects progressive disease may help more than pharmacological intervention.
- Remember the contribution of open and sensitive communication to successful symptom control, eliciting patients' concerns and involving patients in decision-making.
- Attend to detail at every stage of assessment and management.
- Consider seeking help from the multidisciplinary team, including physiotherapists, psychologists, and chaplains.
- Never 'give up'; there are invariably further strategies that can be tried.

Barriers to symptom control

There is mounting evidence that the symptom control needs of patients with advanced respiratory disease are not being met.[2, 3] This is particularly true for those with benign CRD who, compared to patients with LC:
- are more likely to suffer from uncontrolled symptoms
- experience morbidity over a longer period of time
- receive fewer medications to control symptoms.

A number of factors contribute to inadequate symptom control in non-malignant disease:
- Clinicians erroneously perceive that providing symptom control is inconsistent with disease-modifying treatment and tantamount to 'giving up'.
- Staff lack experience in providing symptom control in benign CRD—palliative care specialists mostly care for those with cancer and respiratory specialists are more familiar with disease-modifying treatment.
- Prescribers are concerned about the potential adverse effects of medication, such as respiratory depression from opioids or anxiolytics.
- Professionals and patients experience therapeutic nihilism, believing that there is no treatment for a number of symptoms, such as fatigue.
- There is a failure to appreciate the importance of a focus on quality of life in benign disease, due to under-recognition of the poor prognosis and unpredictable trajectory.
- Professionals and patients may perceive that smoking-induced CRD is self-inflicted, rendering such patients less eligible for or deserving of measures to improve quality of life.
- The evidence base is inadequate, most research on symptom control being carried out in those with cancer, and often focusing on the physical rather than psychological dimension.

The key to overcoming these barriers lies in the education of all health-care professionals involved in the care of patients with advanced respiratory disease. Such education must focus on:
- mixed management models of care, combining disease-modifying treatment with symptom control interventions
- sharing of evidence-based best practice and knowledge between disciplines, in particular between respiratory and palliative care specialists.

References

1. Edmonds P, Karlsen S, Khan S, et al. (2001) A comparison of the palliative care needs of patients dying from chronic respiratory diseases and lung cancer. *Palliat Med*; 15: 287–295.
2. Au D, Udris E, Fihn S et al. (2006) Differences in health utilization at the end of life among patients with chronic obstructive pulmonary disease and patients with lung cancer. *Arch Intern Med*; 166: 326–331.
3. Habraken J, Riet G, Gore J et al. (2009) Health-related quality of life in end-stage COPD and lung cancer patients. *J Pain Sy Manage*; 37 (6): 973–981.

Pain in respiratory disease

Definitions

- 'Pain is an unpleasant sensory and emotional experience associated with actual or potential tissue damage, or described in terms of such damage.'[1]
- 'Nociception' is the perception of a painful stimulus by the nervous system. Pain is the personal experience of this.
- 'Total pain' is a term that encompasses the multidimensional nature of pain. Physical, psychological, social, and spiritual elements all contribute to patients' suffering.

Pain is a psychosomatic phenomenon affected by mood, morale, and the meaning the pain has for the patient.

Prevalence

Pain is a common symptom experienced by the majority of patients with advanced respiratory disease. Prevalence data vary widely due to heterogeneity of study populations and outcomes. It is, however, apparent that:

- lung cancer is one of the most primary neoplasms to cause pain, and approximately three-quarters of those with incurable disease suffer from this symptom
- non-malignant CRD is also associated with pain in one- to two-thirds of patients, and the pain in such patients is particularly under-assessed and inadequately managed.

Causes

Pain in LC is usually due to the disease itself. Pain in CRD is more likely to be due to complications of the disease or concurrent morbidity.

Primary respiratory disease

- Local malignant invasion of primary lung cancer such as:
  - apical Pancoast's tumour infiltrating brachial plexus
  - peripheral disease infiltrating pleura, ribs, and chest wall
  - central disease invading mediastinum
- Metastatic spread of malignancy to bone, brain, liver etc.
- Paraneoplastic syndromes such as myositis and peripheral neuropathy.

Complications of respiratory disease

- Chest infection causing pleuritis or tracheobronchitis.
- Rib fracture, costochondritis, and muscle sprain secondary to cough.
- Diaphragmatic and intercostal muscle fatigue.
- Pulmonary embolism.
- Pneumothorax.
- Pleural effusion.
- Hypertrophic pulmonary osteoarthropathy.

Treatment of respiratory disease

- Steroid-induced osteoporosis causing vertebral crush fractures.
- Post-thoracotomy pain.
- Peripheral neuropathy caused by chemotherapy such as cisplatin.

Concurrent morbidity
- Osteoarthritis.
- Cardiovascular disease.
- Oesophagitis.
- Constipation.
- Intercostal radiculopathy.
- Herpes zoster infection.

Most pain in advanced respiratory disease is predominantly felt in the chest. This is particularly true for pain that is caused by the primary respiratory disease or a complication of that disease.

Consequences

The consequences of living with uncontrolled pain can be significant. Restriction of chest wall movement and reduction in overall mobility can cause a number of physical sequelae that contribute to morbidity and indeed mortality. The psychosocial consequences of pain are also considerable and can have a profoundly negative impact on carers and family, as well as on the patient.

Table 6.1 Potential consequences of uncontrolled pain

Physical	Psychosocial
• Difficulty coughing	• Anxiety and depression
• Hypoventilation	• Reduced social performance
• Lung atelectasis	• Inability to work
• Chest infection	• Social isolation
• Pressure sores	• Financial difficulties
• Deconditioning	• Strained relationships
• Venous thromboembolism	

Reference

1. IASP Task Force on Taxonomy, edited by Merskey H, Bogduk, N (1994) *Classification of Chronic Pain, 2nd edition*, IASP Press, Seattle.

Assessment of pain

The purpose of assessing a patient's pain is to determine the most likely cause of the symptom. Knowledge of the cause of pain facilitates effective pain management because it allows:
- treatment of any reversible underlying cause of the symptom
- selection of the most appropriate analgesic regimen.

Accurate assessment of a patient's pain is a vital skill that is underpinned by a number of important principles:
- Always believe the patient's complaint of pain. 'Pain is what a patient says it is.'
- Most patients have more than one pain; each pain must be assessed individually and prioritized.
- Evaluation of psychosocial and spiritual factors is as important as assessment of the physical symptom.
- Assessment of pain is rarely a one-off event and often requires multiple consultations over a period of time.

History

Pain is a subjective and complex experience and a detailed history of the symptom is the key to its assessment. It is important to gain the patient's confidence and establish a trusting relationship. Good communication skills also improve the quality of the pain history and include active listening, open questioning, and summarizing of information received.

Details of the pain itself must be established, particularly its site, severity, character, temporal pattern, and associated symptoms. The mnemonic SOCRATES is widely used as a tool to aid recall of these factors (see Figure 6.1). Other important information includes:
- Management of pain so far:
  - current and past medication including dose, route, response, side effects, and reason for discontinuation
  - previous medical consultations
  - non-pharmacological treatments.
- Consequences of the pain:
  - psychological state
  - impact on ADLs and social functioning.
- Patient's understanding of the meaning of the pain:
  - likely cause of the symptom
  - implications for the patient.

This latter factor can be one of the most revealing areas of enquiry:
- Patients can be remarkably accurate in appraising the cause of pain; they have first-hand knowledge of the characteristics of the symptom and a vested interest in determining its cause.
- Mistaken beliefs as to the cause and implications of the symptom can hinder control of pain and can be relatively easily corrected.

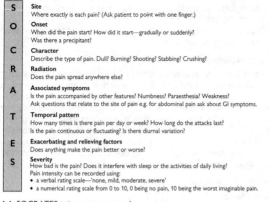

S	**Site** Where exactly is each pain? (Ask patient to point with one finger.)
O	**Onset** When did the pain start? How did it start—gradually or suddenly? Was there a precipitant?
C	**Character** Describe the type of pain. Dull? Burning? Shooting? Stabbing? Crushing?
R	**Radiation** Does the pain spread anywhere else?
A	**Associated symptoms** Is the pain accompanied by other features? Numbness? Paraesthesia? Weakness? Ask questions that relate to the site of pain e.g. for abdominal pain ask about GI symptoms.
T	**Temporal pattern** How many times is there pain per day or week? How long do the attacks last? Is the pain continuous or fluctuating? Is there diurnal variation?
E	**Exacerbating and relieving factors** Does anything make the pain better or worse?
S	**Severity** How bad is the pain? Does it interfere with sleep or the activities of daily living? Pain intensity can be recorded using: • a verbal rating scale—'none, mild, moderate, severe' • a numerical rating scale from 0 to 10, 0 being no pain, 10 being the worst imaginable pain.

Fig. 6.1 SOCRATES pain assessment tool.

DS was a 61-year-old lady with stage 3b NSCLC who had been treated with chemotherapy and radiotherapy 6 months ago. She was admitted to hospital in a state of distress, complaining of severe epigastric pain. It was considered that the pain was likely to be due to gastritis secondary to the use of a non-steroidal anti-inflammatory drug. However, the pain did not resolve after commencing the proton pump inhibitor, omeprazole. She subsequently underwent a gastroscopy that confirmed the presence of gastritis. The pain persisted. Two days later she was asked 'What do you think might be causing this pain?' She responded, 'I know that you think there is an irritation in my stomach, but I'm afraid that this pain means that the cancer has spread.' She was reassured strongly that there was no evidence of disease progression on a recent chest X-ray. The epigastric pain resolved that day.

Examination

- Pay particular attention to the exact site of pain (facilitated by the patient pointing with one finger to the site of worst pain on exposed body part).
- Palpate at the site of pain to elicit tenderness or palpate abnormal swellings, areas of muscle spasm etc.
- Undertake a full neurological examination of the affected area, particularly in the presence of neck or back pain.
- Observe for the degree of functional impairment while moving in and out of a chair, undressing etc.
- Remember general observation of mood, wincing, grimacing etc.

Abnormal sensory signs include:
- paraesthesia—any abnormal sensation, whether spontaneous or evoked
- analgesia—an absence of pain in response to a stimulus that would normally be painful

- hyperalgesia—an increased painful response to a stimulus that would normally be painful
- allodynia—pain caused by a stimulus, such as a light touch, that should not normally provoke pain.

Investigations

These do not form an important part of the clinical evaluation of pain and serve mainly to confirm or refute the clinical diagnosis of the cause of pain. Computerized tomography (CT), magnetic resonance imaging (MRI), positron emission tomography (PET), and radio-isotope scanning can be used to assess the site and extent of malignant disease. MRI is of value in appraising skeletal or soft tissue pathology and evaluating potential neurological involvement e.g. brachial plexus disease. Thoracic ultrasound (USS) and contrast-enhanced CT scanning can accurately demonstrate pleural pathology.

Outcomes of assessment

Cause of pain

By the end of the pain assessment the intention is to have determined the most likely cause of the pain(s) or a short differential diagnosis. This greatly facilitates pain management by allowing the treatment of reversible causes of pain and aiding analgesic selection.

Type of pain

In addition, the assessment can allow the type of pain to be characterized (see Table 6.2). Knowledge of the likely pain type can help determine the most likely cause of pain and can aid selection of the most appropriate analgesic. The type of pain can be described according to:

- Pathophysiology:
  - nociceptive pain—following somatic or visceral tissue damage and conducted by a normal nervous system
  - neuropathic pain—either following nerve injury or compression.
- Temporal pattern:
  - acute pain—following an event that would be expected to cause pain such as a pathological fracture
  - chronic pain—a persistent pain that requires continual analgesia
  - breakthrough pain—intermittent exacerbations of pain otherwise well controlled with appropriate doses of analgesia
  - incident pain—absent at rest and brought on by a particular movement such as walking or coughing.
- Response to opioids:
  - opioid-responsive—a good response to opioids, without significant or uncontrollable adverse effects
  - partially opioid-responsive—some response, but pain incompletely controlled and increase in opioid dose limited by adverse effects
  - poorly opioid-responsive—little/no response to opioid treatment.

Table 6.2 Characteristics of different pain types

Pain type	Examples	Typical clinical features
Nociceptive somatic	Osteoporotic vertebral fracture Rib fracture Muscle injury	Sometimes described as 'aching' 'stabbing' or 'throbbing' in nature and may be worse on movement.
Nociceptive visceral	Liver capsule pain secondary to hepatic metastases from lung cancer Bowel colic secondary to consipation	'Gnawing' or 'cramping' character, sometimes 'sharp' or 'throbbing' when solid organ or capsule involved
Neuropathic	Spinal nerve root compression Post thoracotomy pain	'Burning' 'tingling' or 'deep aching' quality. Occasionally lancinating 'like an electric shock'. Can be associated with abnormal sensations such as allodynia. Often partially or poorly responsive to strong opioids

Mr WS was a 63-year-old gentleman with severe COPD. He presented in some distress with a 48-hour history of increasing breathlessness and a new chest pain that was worse on inspiration, and he was immediately admitted to hospital for evaluation and treatment of a suspected pulmonary embolus. A detailed pain history established that the pain had started after he had stumbled at home and fallen against a door. The pain was 'stabbing' in nature and was worse when he moved or took a deep breath, and it radiated between his back and a point near his left nipple. He had noticed that even his shirt rubbing on the skin there was uncomfortable. On examination, there was focal, mid-thoracic spinal tenderness and a band of allodynia across his left chest.

The pain was classified as an acute, incident, thoracic bone pain with associated acute neuropathic pain in the T6 dermatome. A steroid-induced osteoporotic vertebral collapse with nerve root compression was considered to be the most likely cause of the pain and the diagnosis was confirmed by an MRI scan. He could not tolerate non-steroidal anti-inflammatory drugs or strong opioids, and a trial of gabapentin was ineffective. A vertebroplasty was performed under local anaesthetic. He made an uneventful recovery, mild residual pain being fully controlled by regular paracetamol.

This case demonstrates the importance of a detailed pain assessment. This can help determine the *type* of pain, which in turn facilitates diagnosis of the underlying *cause* of pain. Once the cause is known, its reversal can lead to highly effective pain relief.

Overview of pain management

Treatment of reversible causes

The most effective method of treating any symptom is to reverse the underlying cause. Pain is no exception to this principle and examples include:

- treatment of infection-induced pleuritic pain with antibiotics
- relief of dyspepsia secondary to gastritis with a proton pump inhibitor
- surgical fixation of a malignant pathological bone fracture
- use of appropriate diet and laxatives to treat bowel colic secondary to constipation.

Oral analgesia

The World Health Organization guidelines for the use of analgesic drugs are recommended and used worldwide. Although developed initially for use in cancer pain, they provide a useful framework for all chronic pain irrespective of cause. The use of oral analgesics is described in detail on 📖 pp. 98–110.

The principles of analgesic use are as follows:

- Use a three-step ladder (Figure 6.2). Start with step 1, reassess after 24 hours, and move up the ladder if pain remains inadequately controlled.
- Prescribe regular analgesia. This is more effective than 'as needed' analgesia, taken only when the pain is present.
- In addition, prescribe 'as needed' medication for breakthrough pain i.e. pain that breaks through despite the regular analgesic.
- Use the oral route. If inadequate analgesia is achieved, consider a higher dose or an alternative analgesic rather than altering the route. Other than a faster onset of action, an equianalgesic parenteral dose is usually no more effective in patients with unimpaired absorption of oral drugs.
- Monitor frequently to assess for efficacy or adverse effects. Adjust drug dose or type as needed and actively treat adverse effects.

Non-pharmacological approaches

Oral analgesics are the primary method of pain control. Non-drug approaches can be combined with oral analgesia as an adjunct, particularly if suboptimal analgesia has been achieved. The multidimensional nature of pain is reflected in the use of the following holistic and patient-centred approaches:

- Psychological interventions. Useful techniques include:
  - cognitive behavioural therapy—aiming to change maladaptive thoughts and behaviours
  - relaxation—such as passive relaxation (focusing attention on sensations of warmth and decreased tension around the body) and progressive muscular relaxation (active tensing and relaxing of muscles)
  - imagery/distraction techniques—the patient can, for example, imagine a place or activity where he/she felt most safe and secure and then can focus on this, utilizing all the senses.
- Radiotherapy can be considered in pain caused by malignant disease.

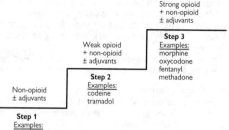

Opioids are agonists at endogenous opioid receptors, such as the mu receptor, producing 'morphine-like' activity.
Adjuvants are additional drugs that can be used as part of pain management, such as secondary analgesics (e.g. gabapentin for neuropathic pain) and drugs to control analgesic adverse effects.

Fig. 6.2 World Health Organization three-step analgesic ladder.
(Adapted from WHO (1996) Cancer pain relief: with a guide to opioid availability, 2nd edn. Geneva: WHO).

A narrative for progressive muscle relaxation could go as follows:[1]
'I wonder if you could tense up every muscle in your body… that's it, squeeze in the muscles… hold it, and then just let it go… once more, tense up your muscles… make them very tight and tense, hold it, hold it… and then breathe out, and let your muscles relax, just let them go… Now, as your body begins to feel more and more relaxed, clench your jaw, squeeze it tight, clench it, then let it go… now open your mouth wide, as wide as it will go, stick out your tongue, stick it way out, hold it, then let it go. Feel your head becoming more and more relaxed, as it sinks down into the pillow, allowing all the tension and tightness to drift out of it. Now I wonder if you can lift up your shoulders, lift them up, up to your ears, hold them there squeezing them tightly, squeeze and then let them drop down, just let them go… and then once more, lift them up… hold it… then let them go… as you feel all the tightness and tension in your shoulders begin to drain away… Now I wonder if you can clench your hands into fists, make a tight fist as your whole arm tightens, tense your arms as you squeeze your fingers tighter and tighter… and now just let them go, once more make a fist, a tight fist, hold it, and then let it go…'

There is little evidence to support the efficacy of the following techniques, but they can be highly effective for some individuals and, at worst, do not appear to cause significant harm:

- Transcutaneous electrical nerve stimulation (TENS)—indications for the treatment of chest pain could include:
  - post-thoracotomy pain (electrodes on either side of scar)
  - rib fracture or metastasis (electrodes on either side of affected rib)

- neuropathic pain from intercostal radiculopathy or post-herpetic neuralgia (electrodes above or across affected dermatome)
- Acupuncture—this appears to be most useful for pain due to muscle spasm, such as injury following prolonged coughing, and for post-thoracotomy pain.
- Complementary therapies—these include massage, reflexology, aromatherapy, and creative therapies such as art and music therapy.

Anaesthetic techniques

These techniques are used when a patient fails to gain adequate pain control with systemic analgesia. They can be considered as the fourth and highest step on the analgesic ladder.

- Spinal analgesia is the most frequently used anaesthetic technique:
  - Drugs are injected through either an epidural or, preferably, subarachnoid (intrathecal) catheter.
  - Morphine is the most widely used spinal analgesic, being the least lipid soluble, and it is often combined with a local anaesthetic (e.g. bupivicaine) and α_2-adrenergic agonist (e.g. clonidine).
  - In advanced respiratory disease, the main roles for spinal analgesia are to treat uncontrolled pain from vertebral compression fractures or rib fractures, or to control intractable cancer pain.
- Local anaesthetic or neurolytic nerve blocks tend to be reserved for patients in whom spinal analgesia is contraindicated:
  - Neurolytic intercostal nerve blocks or paravertebral blocks can be used in intractable chest wall pain, such as that caused by malignant chest wall invasion.
  - Before proceeding with neurolysis, a prognostic local anaesthetic block should be used to determine whether neurolysis is likely to be effective.
  - Cingulotomy and cervical cordotomy are occasionally used in specialist centres, particularly for uncontrolled chest pain related to mesothelioma.

Reference

1. Breitbart W, Payne D, Passik S (2005) Psychological and psychiatric interventions in pain control. In: Doyle D, Hanks G, Cherny N, Calman K (eds.), *Oxford Textbook of Palliative Medicine*, 3rd edition. Oxford University Press, Oxford, pp424–438.

Non-opioid analgesia

Paracetamol and non-steroidal anti-inflammatory drugs (NSAIDs) are the principal non-opioid analgesics. They can be used alone in step 1 of the WHO ladder (Figure 6.2) and can also be effective in combination with opioids in steps 2 and 3.

Paracetamol

- Paracetamol is a synthetic non-opioid analgesic that acts centrally, inhibiting brain cyclo-oxygenase and nitric oxide synthetase.
- It has a high oral bioavailability (90% after 1g paracetamol); onset of analgesia occurs in 15–30 minutes and analgesia lasts 4–6 hours.
- The usual route of administration is oral, although it can be given intravenously and rectally if the oral route is not available. Intravenous paracetamol has an earlier onset and longer duration of action than oral paracetamol.
- Adverse effects are very rare and occur in less than 0.1% of patients. However, patients who are elderly and poorly nourished have lower glutathione stores and are more susceptible to hepatic toxicity.
- Concurrent use of 5HT3 receptor antagonists with paracetamol may completely block the analgesic effect of the drug.
- Dispersible paracetamol tablets have a high sodium content and should be avoided in patients with hypertension or renal impairment.
- A small proportion of patients who experience bronchospasm with NSAIDs or aspirin (probably less than 2%) may also develop bronchospasm following paracetamol. The reaction to paracetamol is less severe than to NSAIDs.

Recommendations in advanced respiratory disease:
- Prescribe regular oral paracetamol 1g qds as the first step in the management of chronic pain.
- If there has been no definite benefit within 48 hours, stop the drug.
- When a strong opioid is added to paracetamol (WHO ladder step 3) and pain control is good, review the need for paracetamol by stopping it, only reinstating it if the pain returns.
- Patients with a history of NSAID- or aspirin-induced bronchospasm should take a test dose of 250mg paracetamol and be observed for a few hours before commencing regular full-dose paracetamol.

Formulations:
- Tablets, 500mg.
- Dispersible tablets, 500mg.
- Capsules, 500mg.
- Oral suspension, 120mg/5mL, 250mg/5mL.
- Suppositories, 60mg, 125mg, 250mg, 500mg.
- Intravenous infusion, 10mg/mL.

NSAIDs

NSAIDs inhibit the enzyme cyclo-oxgenase, thereby reducing the production of pro-inflammatory prostaglandins. They can be categorized according to their selectivity for COX-1 and COX-2 isoforms:

- preferential COX-1 inhibition—indometacin, ketorolac
- non-selective—ibuprofen, naproxen, flurbiprofen
- preferential COX-2 inhibition—diclofenac, celecoxib, meloxicam
- selective COX-2 inhibitors—parecoxib, valdecoxib, etoricoxib.

Adverse effects

NSAIDs are highly effective analgesics, particularly for musculoskeletal pain. However, their use is hindered by their adverse effect profile as detailed in Table 6.3. Potentially serious complications include:

- gastroduodenal toxicity such as ulceration
- acute bronchospasm
- thrombotic events such as MI or CVA
- anti-platelet action with resultant risk of bleeding
- renal impairment.

Route of administration

Oral administration, if available, is preferred. There is no evidence for therapeutic advantage from rectal or parenteral preparations.

There is increasing evidence for the efficacy of topical NSAIDs in chronic musculoskeletal pain. In the UK, the National Institute for Health and Clinical Excellence (NICE) has recommended that because of their favourable safety profile, topical NSAIDs should be used in preference to oral NSAIDs for pain related to osteoarthritis. Topical NSAIDs offer:

- enhanced local delivery of the drug to affected tissues
- significantly fewer adverse effects than oral NSAIDs due to low systemic absorption (of 3–5%)
- benefit from rubbing the painful area, possibly contributing to the significant placebo effect.

Recommendations in advanced respiratory disease:
- First-line: for musculoskeletal pain or for other pains associated with inflammation, such as pleurisy, prescribe ibuprofen 400mg tds po.
- Second-line: consider using naproxen 250–500mg bd po.
- Prescribe a proton pump inhibitor concurrently, such as omeprazole 20mg od po.
- Avoid long-term prescription of oral NSAIDs and use for the shortest period of time necessary to control symptoms.
- Prescribe topical NSAIDs for patients with localized superficial muscular pain, costochondritis, or osteoarthritis.
- Use NSAIDs with caution in patients with asthma and COPD patients with significant bronchospasm, and give a test dose under medical supervision.

Formulations of ibuprofen:
- Tablets, 200mg, 400mg, 600mg.
- Oral suspension or syrup, 100mg/5mL.
- Topical forte gel, ibuprofen 10% (Ibugel® Forte).

Formulations of naproxen:
- Tablets, 250mg, 500mg.
- Tablets e/c, 250mg, 375mg, 500mg.

Table 6.3 Adverse effects of NSAIDs

Adverse effect	Comments
Gastroduodenal toxicity	• Lowest risk with coxibs (risk is less than 50% non-selective drugs), ibuprofen and diclofenac. • Risk factors particularly prevalent in advanced respiratory disease include age >65 years, serious co-morbidity, concurrent use of corticosteroid, aspirin, anticoagulant or SSRI.
Acute bronchospasm	• Prevalence is ~20% in adult population and 5% in children. • Typically occurs 0.5-3hrs after ingestion of tablet. • Cross-sensitivity between NSAIDs is high (>90%). • No evidence that COPD increases the risk of sensitivity to NSAIDs, but pragmatic approach is to use NSAIDs with caution in patients with bronchospasm element to disease. • Celecoxib least likely to cause bronchospasm, but avoid because of risk of thrombotic events. • Interestingly, in *population* terms, NSAID use is associated with improved FEV_1, possibly due to anti-inflammatory effect.
Thrombotic cardiovascular events	• Coxibs confer the greatest risk of events such as MI or CVA; most NSAIDs increase risk slightly. • Low dose ibuprofen <1200mg/day and naproxen appear to be safest. • Advanced respiratory disease is a risk factor for thrombotic events, so avoid use of coxibs.
Antiplatelet action	• Aspirin causes irreversible platelet dysfunction, most NSAIDs cause reversible dysfunction, diclofenac and coxibs do not alter function. • Risk of bleeding increased in advanced respiratory disease as patients may require anticoagulation (increased VTE prevalence) or may be taking gastric irritant drugs such as corticosteroids, SSRIs.
Renal impairment	• Cause salt/water retention and can impair renal function, contributing to overall morbidity (eg worsening of cor pulmonale). • Risk factors include chronic renal disease, hypovolaemia and concurrent use of loop diuretics. • Renal risks of NSAIDs are similar, therefore not a factor in determining choice of drug.

Opioid analgesia

Opiates are naturally-occurring opium alkaloids, such as morphine and codeine, and their semi-synthetic derivatives, such as oxycodone and hydromorphone. **Opioids** are fully synthetic drugs with a morphine-like action on the body, such as tramadol, fentanyl, and methadone.

Codeine

- Codeine (methylmorphine) is a naturally-occurring weak opiate that acts mostly through demethylation to morphine by cytochrome P450 CYP2D6. Approximately 7% of Caucasians lack CYP2D6 activity, and in these individuals codeine has a much reduced analgesic effect. Fluoxetine and paroxetine inhibit CYP2D6 and reduce the efficacy of codeine.
- Codeine has approximately one-tenth of the potency of morphine. The usual oral dose is 30–60mg qds and the duration of action of each dose is 4–6 hours.
- There is good evidence that compound preparations containing codeine and paracetamol are more effective than paracetamol alone. Co-codamol 8/500 and 30/500 contain paracetamol 500mg with codeine 8mg and 30mg respectively.
- Codeine causes significant constipation that is greater than an equivalent dose of morphine, and laxatives should be prescribed when the drug is used regularly.

Dihydrocodeine

- Dihydrocodeine is a semi-synthetic analogue of codeine that, unlike codeine, is an active drug rather than a pro-drug. Poor CYP2D6 activity does not appear to impact on the efficacy of dihydrocodeine.
- It is equipotent to oral codeine, but appears to have a narrower therapeutic index leading to more adverse effects at higher doses.

Tramadol

- Tramadol is a moderately strong synthetic analgesic that has both opioid and non-opioid properties. It has a high affinity for μ, δ, and κ opioid receptors, stimulates 5HT release, and inhibits pre-synaptic uptake of 5HT and NA.
- By mouth, it has one-fifth of the potency of morphine and can therefore be considered as double-strength codeine. The usual oral dose is 50–100mg qds and the duration of action of each dose is 4–9 hours.
- It causes less respiratory depression and constipation than equi-analgesic doses of morphine.
- The analgesic effect of tramadol is reduced by ondansetron and possibly other 5HT3 antagonists. Potentially lethal serotonin toxicity can occur when used in combination with other drugs that increase central 5HT levels, such as SSRIs.

Morphine

- Morphine is the strong opiate of choice for the management of moderate to severe chronic pain in advanced respiratory disease. It is used in step 3 of the WHO analgesic ladder, often in combination with non-opioid and adjuvant drugs.
- It is a μ-opioid receptor agonist and is metabolized to M3G and M6G, which are renally excreted. M6G is an active metabolite that can accumulate in renal failure and lead to opioid toxicity.

Starting a patient on oral morphine

- Consider using morphine when a patient is still in pain despite use of a weak opioid and a non-opioid.
- Commence a regular 4-hourly dose of morphine, with the same dose available for prn use:
  - Commence morphine immediate release (IR) 5mg 4-hourly if previously taking 240mg codeine/24 hours (total 30mg morphine/24 hours, 240mg codeine being equivalent to ~24mg morphine).
  - Commence morphine IR 10mg 4-hourly if previously taking 400mg tramadol/24 hours (total 60mg morphine/24 hours, 400mg tramadol being equivalent to ~80mg morphine).
- After 1–2 days recalculate the dose of morphine IR based on total morphine requirement in last 24 hours (both regular and prn).
- When the morphine IR dose is stable, replace it with morphine modified release (MR), prescribed 12-hourly (or daily if a 24-hour formulation). Calculate the 12-hourly morphine MR dose by adding all the morphine IR doses in the previous 24 hours, and divide by 2.
- Continue to prescribe morphine IR for prn use, at a dose of one-sixth of the total morphine dose over 24 hours. The prn dose should be increased when the 24-hour dose increases.
- Warn patients about constipation and prescribe a laxative routinely.
- Explain the possibility of initial drowsiness and nausea. Prescribe an anti-emetic for prn or regular use in the first week, such as haloperidol 1.5mg bd po prn.
- Reassess regularly to evaluate pain control and adverse effects.

Mrs G was a 63-year-old lady with COPD and NSCLC. She developed severe right-sided chest pain that only responded partially to co-codamol 30/500 8 tablets/day. She was converted to paracetamol and morphine IR 5mg 4-hourly and prn. After 24 hours she had used a total of 65mg regular and prn morphine. She was converted to morphine IR 10mg 4-hourly with the same dose for prn use. During the next 24 hours she only required one prn dose, and was then converted to morphine MR 30mg bd with morphine IR 10mg prn for breakthrough pain.

Examples of formulations of morphine IR for 4-hourly use:
- Oral solution, 10mg/5mL (Oramorph®).
- Concentrated oral solution, 100mg/5mL (Oramorph®).
- Tablets, 10mg, 20mg, 50mg (Sevredol®).

Examples of formulations of morphine MR for 12-hourly use (MST Continus®):
- Tablets, 5mg, 10mg, 15mg, 30mg, 60mg, 100mg, 200mg.
- Oral suspension, 20mg, 30mg, 60mg, 100mg, 200mg/sachet.

- Subcutaneous morphine can be used when the oral route is not available. It is twice as potent as oral morphine.
- Adverse effects of morphine are detailed in Table 6.4. Nausea and vomiting, mild drowsiness, and unsteadiness are relatively common initial effects that tend to resolve within the first week of morphine administration. Tolerance to the constipating effect of morphine does not develop, however, and long-term laxatives are usually necessary.

Pain is a physiological antagonist to the respiratory depressant effect of strong opioids.

- When started at a low dose and carefully titrated upwards, morphine does not cause clinically important respiratory depression in patients with pain.
- Significant respiratory depression can occur in patients who are opioid-naïve and are without pain (or with short-lived pain that then subsides, such as post-operatively), particularly if the medication is given parenterally with faster absorption and higher peak concentration. This, in combination with high profile court cases in which doctors have been tried for murder (and the doctrine of double-effect has been used as a successful defence), has led to an entrenched societal misconception that morphine can kill even when used for symptom control.
- Large safety studies have been carried out in cancer patients. Numerous studies involving opioid use for pain and dyspnoea in patients with COPD have never revealed clinically significant respiratory depression but they have, to date, been inadequately powered to detect rare but serious adverse effects.
- In the absence of definitive safety data, care is needed when using morphine in advanced respiratory disease associated with respiratory failure.

Diamorphine
- Diamorphine (di-acetylmorphine, heroin) is considered to be a pro-drug for morphine. Subcutaneous diamorphine is three times more potent than oral morphine.
- It has no clinical advantage over morphine, other than being much more water-soluble. Therefore, in countries where it is available, it is the strong opioid of choice for parenteral use when high doses are needed, as it can be given in a smaller volume.

Table 6.4 Adverse effects of morphine

Effect	Comments	Management
Nausea	Opioid effect on chemoreceptor trigger zone, tolerance develops	Haloperidol 1.5mg bd Consider opioid switch if persists
Constipation	Persistent symptom, laxative invariably needed	See pp. 132–133 for laxative details
Gastric stasis	Early satiety, hiccup, anorexia, vomiting	Metoclopramide 10mg qds
Dry mouth	Tends to persist	Frequent sips of water Saliva substitutes
Sedation	Drowsiness, tolerance usually develops	Reduce opioid dose Look for other causes if persists
Vestibular stimulation	Vertigo, 'unsteadiness', movement induced nausea and vomiting	Cyclizine 25-50mg tds Consider opioid switch
Neurotoxicity	Agitated delirium, hallucinations, myoclonus, hyperalgesia	Reduce opioid dose Consider opioid switch
Pruritis	Whole body itch, does not respond to antihistamines	Ondansetron 8mg po bd

Alternative strong opioids

Although morphine is the strong opioid of choice, alternative opioids may be used in the following situations:
- poor response to morphine plus adjuvant drugs
- unacceptable adverse effects from morphine
- transdermal route preferable
- moderate to severe renal impairment.

Before switching to an alternative opioid, consider the following:
- The pain may be poorly opioid responsive, such as neuropathic pain, and may require alternative interventions rather than opioid switching (see pp. 108–110).
- Adverse effects could be controlled by reducing the morphine dose and prescribing medication to treat the adverse effects, such as haloperidol for nausea or hallucinations.

The characteristics of alternative strong opioids are detailed in Table 6.5. Seek specialist advice if unfamiliar with a drug. Take particular care with fentanyl and methadone in respiratory disease (see p. 106).

Dose conversions between strong opioids (Table 6.5) are approximate. Always err on the side of caution and, if in doubt, convert to a dose under the calculated equivalent. Conversions are particularly likely to be inaccurate when higher doses are involved; it is then safest to give 50% or less of the calculated dose.

Recommendations in advanced respiratory disease:
• Use codeine as the first-line weak opiate for mild to moderate pain.
• Tramadol has a role in patients with severe constipation or type II respiratory failure.
• Morphine is the first-line strong opioid for use in moderate to severe pain. Start with a low dose, titrate carefully, and assess repeatedly.
• Prescribe laxatives. Warn about initial adverse effects, such as nausea, that should settle in the first week, and consider prescribing an anti-emetic for use if needed.
• In patients with type II respiratory failure, commence morphine under medical supervision and if appropriate (not in terminal phase) consider checking arterial blood gases after 24–48 hours.
• Consider opioid switching to oxycodone in patients who cannot tolerate morphine.
• Avoid using the lipophilic and highly protein-bound opioids, fentanyl and methadone, without specialist advice and support.

Warning: lipophilic and highly protein-bound opioids are associated with a risk of respiratory depression occurring with little warning. Cachexia leads to a fall in the volume of distribution and more drug entering the plasma compartment. In addition, increasing pCO_2 causes:
• vasodilatation and increased mobilization of drug from fat to plasma
• reduced plasma protein binding due to acidosis, releasing free drug.

The resulting 'vicious cycle' can occasionally lead to rapid development of opioid toxicity and potentially lethal respiratory depression.

Table 6.5 Comparison of opioids with oral morphine

Drug	Advantages	Disadvantages	Dose conversion example
Codeine (po)	Familiar, avoids 'stigma' of morphine	More constipating, 'ceiling' effect, no analgesic effect in ~1 in 10 Caucasians	Codeine 240mg po ≡ morphine 24mg po
Tramadol (po)	Less constipation and respiratory depression, a potent 'weak' opioid	Risk of seizures or serotonin toxicity	Tramadol 400mg po ≡ morphine 60–80mg po
Diamorphine (sc)	Highly soluble, suitable for high dose parenteral use	Limited availability, only within UK and Belgium	Diamorphine 10mg sc ≡ morphine 30mg po
Oxycodone (po, sc)	Vomiting, hallucinations, pruritis less common, slightly safer in renal impairment	More expensive	Oxycodone 10mg po ≡ morphine 15–20mg Oxycodone 10mg sc ≡ morphine 10mg sc ≡ morphine 20mg po
Fentanyl (TD)	Useful when oral route unavailable, safe in renal failure, less constipating	Cannot be titrated rapidly	Fentanyl patch 25mcg/hr ≡ morphine 60–90mg/24hrs po
Fentanyl (SL/TM)	Rapid onset and short half-life, role in breakthrough pain, safe in renal failure	Expensive, administration requires co-operation	Always start with lowest dose and titrate up (eg Actiq®200mcg lozenge, eg Abstral®100mcg tablet)
Alfentanil (sc)	Short half-life, can be used in syringe driver, safe in renal failure, small volume	Unfamiliar	Alfentanil 1mg sc ≡ diamorphine 10mg sc ≡ morphine 30mg po
Methadone (po)	Role in neuropathic pain, safe in renal failure	Long half-life, danger of accumulation, only commence in specialist unit	Give 3 hourly prn doses 1/30 of previous 24 hr oral morphine dose
Buprenorphine (TD)	Useful when oral route not available, safe in renal failure, less constipating	Skin reactions common, cannot be reversed with naloxone, unfamiliar	Buprenorphine patch 10mcg/hr ≡ morphine 30mg/24hrs po

Dose conversions are only a guide. Always convert cautiously particularly at higher doses. Erroneous conversions can be fatal. Seek specialist advice if unfamiliar with drug.

Key po: oral, sc: subcutaneous, TD: transdermal, SL: sublingual, TM: transmucosal

Difficult pain problems

Opioid poorly responsive pain

Most pain can be controlled with oral analgesics and adjuvant drugs, used in accordance with the WHO ladder (Figure 6.2). Some pain does not, however, respond easily to these approaches and can be complex to manage. Upward titration of the opioid dose may lead to intolerable and/or uncontrollable adverse effects without achieving adequate pain control. There are a number of potential causes of opioid poorly responsive pain that can occur in advanced respiratory disease:

● neuropathic pain
● bone pain and other incident pain
● 'total' pain.

Neuropathic pain

This is pain that is precipitated by either peripheral or central nervous system injury. Possible causes in this patient group include:

● Post-thoracotomy pain caused by surgical damage of peripheral nerves.
● Radicular pain from spinal nerve root damage, such as secondary to osteoarthritis or vertebral/paraspinal malignant disease.
● Herpes zoster infection, triggered, for example, by immunosuppression secondary to corticosteroid use.
● Brachial plexus infiltration by apical lung cancer (Pancoast tumour).
● Chest wall infiltration by mesothelioma causing intercostal nerve injury.

Neuropathic pain typically has a 'burning', 'tingling', or 'deep aching' quality. It can be lancinating 'like an electric shock' and can be associated with abnormal sensations such as allodynia. It is often poorly or only partially responsive to strong opioids.

This type of pain can be responsive to NSAIDs. Consider conversion to an alternative NSAID and maximize opioid dose, whilst actively treating opioid adverse effects. If this fails to achieve adequate pain control, consider the following options in a step-wise approach.

● Anticonvulsant *or* tricyclic antidepressant (TCA):
  • Gabapentin 100mg od, titrated up to tds over 3–6 days, then 300mg od, titrated up to tds over a further week; or amitriptyline 10mg nocte, titrated up to maximum of 50mg nocte.
  • Choose gabapentin if you wish to avoid anti-muscarinic adverse effects.
  • Choose amitripyline if night sedation would be useful, a daily dose preferable, or antidepressant action is required.
● Anticonvulsant *and* TCA:
  • If there is no benefit from first drug, stop and try an alternative drug.
  • If there is incomplete benefit from first drug, add in an alterative drug.
● Corticosteroids:
  • Consider dexamethasone 4–8mg od, particularly if nerve compression is more likely than infiltration.

- Topical lidocaine patch:
  - Lidocaine 5% patch can be effective for superficial, localized pain.
  - Cut matrix patch to size of painful area; up to three patches can be used at a time if area is large.
  - Change patch daily, keeping on for 12 hours out of every 24 hours.
- Opioid switch to methadone:
  - Methadone has NMDA receptor antagonist activity that can reduce the central sensitization that occurs with chronic neuropathic pain.
  - Only commence in a specialist unit (see Table 6.5).
- Spinal or peripheral anaesthetic procedures:
  - See 📖 p. 96.
- Ketamine:
  - This dissociative anaesthetic is a potent NMDA receptor antagonist.
  - It can be effective for neuropathic pain but its use is hindered by a high prevalence of psychotomimetic phenomena including euphoria.
  - Commence on 10–25mg po tds and prn and titrate up to 50mg qds if necessary. Alternatively, administer 'short-burst therapy' by continuous subcutaneous infusion (CSCI), 100mg/24hrs, increased after 24 hours to 300mg/24hrs if not effective, and then to 500mg/24hrs after a further 24 hours if still not effective. Stop 3 days after last dose increment.
  - Unless familiar with the drug, prescribe only with specialist support.

Bone pain and other incident pain

Incident pain is pain that is evoked by specific activities such as moving in bed, walking, coughing, sneezing etc. Its episodic nature means that it is a type of breakthrough pain; in other words a flare of pain occurring on a background of otherwise well-controlled pain.

This type of intermittent pain is difficult to control because, if sufficient analgesia is given to control the pain when it occurs, during the time when the triggering activity is not being performed and the patient is pain free a relative excess of analgesia may lead to adverse effects.

Causes of incident pain in respiratory disease include:
- rib fracture
- rib or vertebral bone metastasis
- muscle sprain
- costochondritis
- pleurisy.

Consider the following management options:
- NSAIDs with gastroprotection, often the most effective approach. Consider switching to an alternative NSAID if pain control is inadequate.
- Single fraction palliative radiotherapy for malignant bone pain.
- Bisphosphonates for malignant bone pain (may also prevent pathological fractures).
- Oral transmucosal fentanyl citrate lozenges or sublingual fentanyl tablets (see Table 6.5) for rapid onset and brief analgesia during time of triggering activity.

'Total pain'

This concept encompasses the physical, psychological, social, and spiritual factors that contribute to this complex, multidimensional, and subjective symptom. When the complaint of pain is more a reflection of the psychological or spiritual turmoil being experienced by a patient, such pain will not respond to morphine. Such pain is sometimes termed 'opioid irrelevant pain'.

Careful communication and exploration of underlying mood, concerns, and expectations will be more effective than a pharmacological approach. Specialist psychological interventions may be needed.

Pain control in renal failure

Management of pain in patients with advanced respiratory disease and concurrent renal impairment can be challenging. A number of commonly used analgesics become unsafe to use. Morphine is converted to active metabolites that are excreted through the renal system. Accumulation of such metabolites in renal impairment can lead to significant opioid toxicity and potential respiratory depression. Furthermore, NSAIDs are contra-indicated. The safest drugs to use at each step of the WHO ladder are as follows:

- Step 1:
  - Paracetamol: 1g qds, reducing to 1g tds when GFR <10mL/min.
- Step 2:
  - Tramadol: 50–100mg qds reducing to 50mg bd when GFR <50mL/min.
- Step 3:
  - Alfentanil subcutaneous infusion: dose unaltered by renal failure.
  - Fentanyl (transdermal, subcutaneous, or transmucosal): titrate to pain
  - Morphine: small doses on prn basis only, when GFR <50mL/min.
  - Methadone oral or subcutaneous infusion: only in specialist unit.

See Table 6.5 for further details.
- Adjuvant drugs:
  - Amitriptyline: use normal dose.
  - Gabapentin: maximum of 300mg/24hrs when GFR <50mL/min.

Fatigue

After breathlessness, fatigue is the most common symptom experienced by patients with advanced respiratory disease. It occurs in more than 50% of patients with advanced lung cancer, and up to 80% of those with COPD. The symptom is multidimensional with physical, affective, and cognitive components.

- Physical:
  - Generalized weakness or limb heaviness.
  - Extreme tiredness.
  - Inability to perform tasks.
- Affective:
  - Low mood.
  - Decreased motivation.
  - Lack of energy.
- Cognitive:
  - Lack of concentration or attention.
  - Difficulty thinking clearly.
  - Poor short-term memory.

Fatigue has a particularly negative impact on quality of life. It can hinder social functioning and ability to self-care, and can lead to a deteriorating cycle of dependence, social isolation, low self-esteem, and depression.

Despite being one of the most prevalent and distressing symptoms, fatigue tends to be neglected by both medical staff and patients. It has traditionally been viewed as an inevitable and unavoidable consequence of advanced disease. However, with diagnosis and active management, fatigue can be ameliorated. It is vital that this important symptom is not ignored.

Causes

The underlying mechanism for fatigue in advanced respiratory disease is unknown, but may involve excess production of pro-inflammatory cytokines (IL6, IL1, and TNF-α) and abnormalities in ATP synthesis. A large number of clinical factors are known to contribute to fatigue as detailed in Table 6.6.

Diagnosis

- Patient reports that tiredness interferes with ability to function and is not relieved by rest.
- Fatigue severity score of ≥5 using an 11-point numerical rating scale ranging from 0 (no fatigue) to 10 (worst fatigue imaginable).

Management

Reverse underlying causes

The key to fatigue management is to search for and correct reversible underlying factors.

Common, treatable contributing causes include:
- depression
- breathlessness
- pain
- sleep disturbance
- drugs e.g. β-blockers
- anaemia
- co-existing infection.

Non-pharmacological approaches

Fatigue causes inactivity, which leads to deconditioning. This, in turn, worsens fatigue. There is high quality evidence that exercise, ranging from gentle exercise at home to formal pulmonary rehabilitation, interrupts this vicious cycle and can significantly improve fatigue.[1] However, in advanced disease, exercise may no longer be appropriate. Patients who still function independently can benefit from a simple explanation as to why keeping reasonably active can be helpful.

As performance status deteriorates, energy conservation techniques become more useful:
- Encourage patients to prioritize and avoid unnecessary activities.
- Discuss adapting tasks so that they require less effort.
- Practise relaxation techniques.

Counselling and support can be helpful too, openly acknowledging the presence and negative impact of the symptom.

Pharmacological approaches

Erythropoetin is the only evidence-based pharmacological treatment for anaemia-related fatigue. However, recent evidence of excess mortality in cancer patients treated with erythropoetin means that use of erythropoetin cannot be recommended for cancer-related fatigue.[2]

Corticosteroids can improve well-being and energy, and there is some evidence from patients with advanced cancer that they can relieve fatigue. However, steroids have considerable adverse effects; proximal myopathy and gastritis-related GI bleeding may increase fatigue. If there has been no improvement in fatigue in 4 weeks, corticosteroids should be stopped.

Central nervous stimulants, such as methylphenidate or modafinil, may have a role, but further research evidence is required before adoption into mainstream practice.

Table 6.6 Factors contributing to fatigue

Clinical correlates	Treatments	Comorbidities
• Depression	• β-blockers	• Anaemia
• Breathlessness	• Opioids	• Infection
• Deconditioning	• Hypnotics	• Cardiac dysfunction
• Sleep disturbance	• Sedative antihistamines	• Adrenal insufficiency
• Cachexia	• Chemotherapy	• Hypothyroidism
• Pain	• Radiotherapy	• Neuromuscular disease

Mrs C is a 72-year-old widow with advanced COPD, who asked for a home visit from her respiratory nurse specialist. She was complaining that, although her breathlessness was in control when she moved slowly, she was getting so tired that she was struggling to make meals and was losing weight. In addition, her daughter had stopped bringing her young grandchildren, as they were making her even more exhausted. She was increasingly spending the whole of her waking day in one chair, over-looking the garden. Recently she had begun to sleep in the chair at night, as she could not gather the energy to go to bed. During the conversation, it became clear that she was afraid that the extreme tiredness was a sign that she was dying.

It was sensitively explained to her that a number of factors were contributing to her fatigue, including deconditioning from inactivity, sleep disturbance from sleeping in a chair, poor nutrition, and low mood due to increasing social isolation and undiscussed fears. Over a number of home visits, she was encouraged to set herself reasonable goals to increase her activity, including walking to the kitchen regularly to make simple, nutritious meals. Her daughter met her specialist nurse, and she began to visit more often and provide support. After one month, Mrs C felt confident enough to take small walks in the garden, and was amazed that her quality of life had improved so much.

References

1. Lacasse Y, Goldstein R, Lasserson TJ, *et al.* (2006) Pulmonary rehabilitation for chronic obstructive pulmonary disease. *Cochrane Database Syst Rev*, CD003793.
2. National Institute for Health and Clinical Evidence Epoetin alfa, epoetin beta darbepoetin alfa for cancer treatment-induced anaemia. NICE technology appraisal guidance 142 May 2008.

Anxiety

Causes

A degree of anxiety is a common consequence of any illness. Advanced respiratory disease is, however, particularly likely to lead to significant anxiety for a number of reasons:

- Breathlessness is both a cause and a consequence of anxiety. This results in a deteriorating vicious circle that can lead to panic (see Figure 6.3).
- The disease trajectory is often associated with sudden and unexpected deteriorations in condition, and this unpredictability can lead to intense fear and uncertainty about the future.
- Patients with advanced respiratory disease are at risk of becoming socially isolated; unexpressed concerns fester and grow.
- Many patients have a poor functional status, a significant proportion becoming housebound, and this can lead to fear of losing independence.
- A number of treatments for respiratory diseases can cause or exacerbate anxiety, such as β_2-agonists and corticosteroids.

Consequences

Patients with respiratory disease who are suffering from anxiety:
- have a significantly worse quality of life
- suffer from more severe dyspnoea
- are more likely to be admitted to hospital
- have poorer outcomes from hospital treatment.

Despite its high prevalence and negative impact, anxiety in patients with respiratory disease is often neglected. There is an expectation that it will be present, which leads to it being ignored. Furthermore, health professionals tend towards therapeutic nihilism, believing that, other than by using potentially harmful drugs such as benzodiazepines, it is not possible to treat. This is not true. A number of interventions have been proven to be effective in the management of anxiety in respiratory disease.

Active screening, diagnosis, and treatment of anxiety has the potential to be one of the most effective approaches to improving the quality of life of patients with advanced respiratory disease.

Diagnosis

Anxiety is a problem that should be actively managed if its severity or duration exceed normal expectations and if it interferes with a patient's ability to function. Screen all patients with advanced respiratory disease for the presence of anxiety, particularly if they are complaining of:
- inability to relax, indecisiveness, irritability, or insomnia
- sweating, tremor, nausea, or panic.

Use a single-item screening question, such as:
- 'Are you feeling very anxious?'
- 'Many people with… (e.g. COPD) find it makes them feel quite worried/frightened/anxious at times. Are you experiencing this too?'

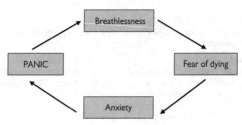

Fig. 6.3 The anxiety-dyspnoea cycle.

- Patients that are anxious tend to be preoccupied with what may happen in the future.
- Patients that are depressed tend to be preoccupied with what has happened in the past.

Management

The mainstay of anxiety management is non-pharmacological. There can be no substitute to giving patients encouragement and time to express their concerns, fears, and expectations. Even in advanced disease it is common for the imagined future to be worse than the likely reality. Listen well and respond with honesty and clarity.

Management of contributing factors

- Dyspnoea—this symptom is inextricably linked with anxiety; the management of one inevitably helps the other.
- Depression—it may be that anxiety symptoms are part of a depressive illness.
- Carer/family anxiety—giving appropriate support to carers can ease the suffering of patients.
- Staff anxiety—this should not be forgotten; anxiety is 'catching' and can impact on the mood and objectivity of healthcare professionals.

Non-pharmacological approaches

Non-drug measures tend to be more effective and better tolerated than pharmacological management of both anxiety and depression.

Pulmonary rehabilitation

There is consistent high-quality evidence that pulmonary rehabilitation can improve both anxiety and depression in patients with COPD, as well as improving breathlessness, fatigue, and quality of life (see 📖 Chapter 5 p. 68 for further details).[1,2]

Cognitive behavioural therapy

CBT has been shown to improve anxiety and depression in advanced COPD (see box)[2].

Other measures

Progressive muscular relaxation, imagery/distraction techniques, and self-hypnosis may all contribute to alleviating anxiety. These approaches require time and cooperation to learn. All techniques need to be practised, and patients derive most benefit if they are taught as early as possible (see 🕮 Chapter 5 p. 73) for further details).

Pharmacological approaches

Despite their 'bad press', benzodiazepines can be useful in the short-term to break the anxiety/dyspnoea cycle and restore sleep. Non-drug approaches should always be used concurrently, and benzodiazepines (BDZ) have a role in helping regain control while waiting for psychological approaches to become effective. The addictive potential is less of a concern when prognosis is short. Consider using the following:

* Diazepam 1–5mg od nocte and prn, long half-life (24–120hrs) giving 'background' symptom control.
* Lorazepam 0.5mg sublingually, rapid onset (5 min onset, time to peak concentration 1hr) useful for prn use at times of acute anxiety.
* Midazolam 2.5mg sc prn or 10–30mg (or more) continuous sc infusion over 24hrs, when oral route not available.

As well as reducing anxiety, BDZ may have a direct effect on reducing dyspnoea (see 🕮 Chapter 5 p. 79), can relax muscle spasm, and raise the seizure threshold, and there is some evidence that clonazepam (250mcg–2mg po od) can be effective in neuropathic pain.

BDZ may cause a paradoxical agitation, or even delirium, in some patients; avoid the classic error of increasing the BDZ dose to control anxiety/agitation in such instances. BDZ have a central respiratory depressant effect and care must therefore be taken in respiratory failure.

A number of non-BDZ drugs have anxiolytic properties:

* Antidepressants with anxiolytic properties include amitriptyline, mirtazapine, paroxetine, and citalopram (see 🕮 pp. 120–121).
* There is limited evidence that buspirone, a non-benzodiazepine anxiolytic, can reduce anxiety in COPD. It takes 2–4 weeks to be effective but may have a role in respiratory failure as it has no respiratory depressant effect. Start at 5mg bd and titrate up the dose every 2–3 days.

Cognitive behavioural therapy for anxiety and panic[4]

The cognitive behavioural approach involves recognizing the way feelings, thoughts, behaviour, and physical sensations can influence each other. A vicious circle can develop (see Figure 6.3) with a spiralling descent into anxiety and panic. A number of helpful and simple cognitive techniques and behavioural experiments can help breathlessness-related anxiety and panic. Consider accessing the services of a trained CBT therapist for specialist help.

1. Psychoeducation: Understand the causes and consequences of hyperventilation; understand that panic does not lead to death; ask the patient to deliberately hyperventilate to demonstrate the associated symptoms and then show the effectiveness of rebreathing with a paper bag.

2. Unhelpful thoughts: Challenge the thoughts that catastrophe and death will occur with more realistic alternatives volunteered by the patient, based on his/her own experience of panic attacks.

3. Breathing control: Encourage learning to relax the abdomen, breathing gently from the diaphragm; practise with two or three diaphragmatic breaths every hour until it becomes easy and natural.

References

1. Withers N, Rudkin S, White R (1999) Anxiety and depression in severe chronic obstructive pulmonary disease: the effects of pulmonary rehabilitation. *J Cardiopul Rehab*;19 (6): 362–365.
2. Coventry PA (2009) Does pulmonary rehabilitation reduce anxiety and depression in chronic obstructive pulmonary disease? *Curr Opin Pulm Medicine*; 15: 143–149.
3. Kunik M, Veazey C, Culley J et al. (2008) COPD education and cognitive behavioural therapy group treatment for clinically significant symptoms of depression and anxiety in COPD patients: a randomised controlled trial. *Psychol Med*; 38 (3): 385–396.
4. Sage N, Sowden M, Chorlton E, Edeleanu A (2008) *CBT for Chronic Illness and Palliative Care: A workbook and toolkit*. John Wiley and Sons Ltd, England.

Depression

Untreated depression, like anxiety, can lead to poor quality of life, worse symptom control, increased admission to hospital, and worse outcomes. Diagnosis and proactive management is of great importance.

Although a significant proportion of patients with advanced respiratory disease become depressed, it is often under-recognized and only one-third of patients with depression receive treatment.

- Medical staff may ignore low mood, considering it to be an 'understandable reaction' to a difficult situation.
- Symptoms such as sleep disturbance, weight loss, and anorexia may be attributed to the underlying disease rather than to depression.
- Patients withhold symptoms of depression as they are embarrassed and fear being stigmatized.
- The focus of medical visits tends to be on disease and physical symptom management.

Diagnosis

An assessment for depression must be undertaken in all patients. A single-item screening tool can be helpful, such as, 'Do you think you have become depressed?'

A number of clinical features can help distinguish a depressive illness from appropriate sadness in patients with advanced disease:

- Anhedonia: lack of interest or pleasure in anything, including things that would normally be enjoyed, such as seeing grandchildren.
- Hopelessness: this may be associated with persistent thoughts of death or suicide.
- Loss of emotion: patients may have a flat affect and be unable to express sad emotions as well as happy ones.
- Low self-esteem: guilty ruminations, loss of confidence, and a sense of worthlessness are particularly relevant when they occur with regard to family and friends.
- Diurnal variation: symptoms are typically worse in the morning rather than later in the day.

Management

Management of contributing factors

Breathlessness, uncontrolled pain, and social isolation are all examples of factors that can contribute to depression.

Non-drug measures

As in the management of anxiety, there is more evidence to support the use of non-drug measures than there is for pharmacological intervention. Both pulmonary rehabilitation and cognitive behavioral therapy can improve depression in patients with chronic lung disease.

The National Institute for Health and Clinical Excellence recommends the use of cognitive behavioural therapy as a first-line intervention for the treatment of mild to moderate depression in patients with a chronic physical health problem[1].

Antidepressants

Antidepressants are recommended for use in patients with moderate to severe depression.

SSRIs (sertraline, citalopram, paroxetine)
* SSRIs are as effective as tricyclic antidepressants, better tolerated, and safer in overdose.
* Avoid fluoxetine in respiratory disease as it may worsen anxiety and there is a greater risk of drug interactions.

Amitriptyline
* Amitriptyline is of particular use when depression is associated with anxiety and insomnia, and/or if the patient is experiencing concurrent neuropathic pain.

Mirtazapine
* Mirtazapine (a noradrenergic and specific serotonergic antidepressant, NaSSA) is a potentially useful antidepressant in patients with respiratory disease.
* It has significant anxiolytic activity (mirtazapine 15mg is equivalent to diazepam 15mg in terms of reducing anxiety), increases appetite, and appears to improve sleep as well as neuropathic pain.
* Start with 15mg at night, and if necessary increase the dose by 15mg every 2 weeks.

Psychostimulants

Antidepressants usually take 2–4 weeks to work. When the prognosis is short, psychostimulants may be considered, as a response can be gained in a small number of days[2].
* Methylphenidate is the best tolerated of the traditional psychostimulants. 10–30% of patients experience anxiety or insomnia, particularly at the start of treatment. Start at 2.5mg bd (on wakening and at lunchtime) and titrate up by increments of 2.5mg bd.
* Modafinil is a novel stimulant that is better tolerated than methylphenidate. There is as yet insufficient evidence to support its use for depression, other than in the context of a clinical trial.

References

1 NICE Depression in adults with a chronic physical health problem. NICE clinical guideline 91, Oct 2009.
2. Candy B, Jones L, Williams R, Tookman A, King M (2008). Psychostimulants for depression. *Cochrane Database Syst Rev*, Issue 2, CD006722.

Insomnia

Sleep disturbance is a common and neglected problem in patients with advanced respiratory disease. Insomnia is a heterogeneous complaint that may involve:
- difficulty initiating sleep
- difficulty maintaining sleep
- early morning wakening
- poor quality or non-restorative sleep.

Prevalence
- Rates vary according to the definition of insomnia.
- Up to 50–60% of patients with chronic lung disease and a similar proportion of those with cancer experience sleep disturbance.
- Using a more strict definition, in the region of 20% of these patients suffer from an insomnia syndrome (see box on p. 123).
- Overall, these prevalence rates are more than twice those experienced by healthy individuals.

Causes
- Direct effect of respiratory disease:
  - cough (can be worse when supine)
  - excess sputum
  - dyspnoea (can be worse when supine)
  - nocturnal oxygen desaturation
  - chest pain.
- Drug treatment:
  - corticosteroids
  - β-adrenoreceptor agonists
  - theophylline.
- Psychological morbidity:
  - anxiety
  - depression.
- Hospitalization:
  - noise or disturbances
  - warm room
  - hospital routines
  - poor sleep hygiene.

Consequences
Insomnia has a highly negative impact on quality of life and results in a number of adverse psychological and physical consequences (Table 6.7).

There is evidence from large epidemiological surveys that insomnia can reduce longevity. Individuals who report sleeping less than 4–6 hours per night have an all-cause mortality that is up to three times greater than those that sleep 7–8 hours per night.

Diagnostic criteria of the insomnia syndrome (ICSD, DSM-IV)
A. Difficulty sleeping characterized by either or both of the following:
- difficulty initiating sleep (30 minutes or more until fall asleep)
- difficulty maintaining sleep (more than 30 minutes of nocturnal awakenings).
B. Sleep disturbance occurs at least three nights per week.
C. Sleep disturbance causes:
- significant impairment of daytime functioning, *or*
- marked distress.

Table 6.7 Consequences of insomnia

Psychological	Physical
• Loss of concentration	• Fatigue, exhaustion
• Poor short term memory	• Muscle aches
• Irritability	• Reduced ability to perform activities
• Depression	• Immune down-regulation
• Anxiety	

Table 6.8 Sleep hygiene methods

Strategy	Techniques
Improve sleep-wake pattern	• Go to bed only when sleepy • Get up at the same time every morning • Regular exercise in morning/afternoon but not evening • Avoid daytime naps • Regular, relaxing pre-sleep routine eg warm bath • Light snack or milky drink before sleep • Avoid going to bed hungry or too full • Avoid excessive liquid intake during evening • Optimise bowel or bladder function
Improve sleep environment	• Aim for dark and quiet bedroom, not too warm or cool • Avoid using bedroom for work, television etc • Only use bed for sleep or sex • Remove clocks and other time cues
Change drug intake	• Avoid caffeine-containing drinks or alcohol • Change diuretic timing for daytime diuresis

Management

Despite being one of the most common symptoms experienced by patients with advanced respiratory disease and having an adverse effect on quality of life, insomnia is a neglected symptom:

- Healthcare professionals tend to view it as an inevitable consequence of advanced disease.
- Patients under-report sleep disturbance.
- Clinicians are understandably reluctant to use drugs such as benzodiazepines, and lack knowledge about effective non-drug approaches.

> Do not rely on patients complaining of insomnia. Clinicians must proactively assess patients for the presence of sleep disturbances.

Treat or remove underlying cause

- Treat infective exacerbations to reduce cough, sputum, dyspnoea etc.
- Avoid use of β-adrenoreceptor agonists before sleep. There is evidence that anti-muscarinic agents can improve sleep.
- Ensure that steroids are never taken after 14:00, as they interfere with normal sleep after this time.

Optimize 'sleep hygiene'

- These simple measures are easily understood by patients and can be a highly effective and entirely safe way of improving sleep (Table 6.8).

Non-pharmacological approaches

- Stimulus control therapy:
  - Aim to re-associate bed/bedroom with rapid sleep onset.
  - Develop good sleep hygiene techniques, including going to bed only when sleepy. If unable to fall asleep or go back to sleep within 15–30 minutes, get out of bed and leave the bedroom, carry out a non-stimulating activity, and return to bed only when sleepy.
- Sleep restriction procedures:
  - Aim to curtail the time in bed awake by creating mild sleep deprivation, which results in more efficient sleep and re-association of bed/bedroom with good sleep.
  - Keep a sleep-wake diary. Time allowed in bed is restricted to the average time asleep or felt to be asleep. Time allowed in bed is increased in small increments of 15–30 minutes every few days. Adhere to a constant wakening time and no daytime naps are allowed.
- Relaxation techniques:
  - Progressive muscular relaxation and visual imagery (see Chapter 5 p. 73) can reduce the arousal that interferes with sleep.
- Cognitive therapy:
  - This aims to challenge unhelpful attitudes and misconceptions about sleep. It is important to reduce both the expectation of and the belief in the need for 'a good night's sleep'.
  - Challenge catastrophizing. Broken sleep is not a catastrophe; a restful night with short periods of sleep will be enough for the body's needs. The need for sleep reduces with age, particularly

when activity levels are low. Recall past experiences of successfully
managing without much sleep.
- Don't 'try' to sleep. Passive acceptance should be encouraged.
- Use mental distraction, particularly if the mind is in 'worry' or
'planning' mode. Reading and story tapes may be helpful.

Pharmacological approaches
- Hypnotics:
  - Benzodiazepine (BDZ) use is limited by the risk of tolerance,
  dependence, daytime sedation, and nocturnal respiratory
  depression. Rebound insomnia can occur on stopping the drug. The
  main role of BDZ lies in short-term use at a crisis point, in order to
  'regain control'.
- Other sedating drugs:
  - Tricyclic antidepressants, mirtazapine, and anti-psychotics all have
  the useful 'side effect' of improving sleep, while avoiding many of
  the risks of BDZ.
- Drugs that improve sleep-wake patterns:
  - Case reports suggest a role for psychostimulants such as
  methylphenidate and modafinil. Alternatively melatonin may be
  prescribed, usually in consultation with a sleep specialist.

Recommendations in advanced respiratory disease:
- Correction of reversible underlying causes, education in sleep
hygiene, and cognitive behavioural non-pharmacological approaches
form the mainstay of insomnia management.
- Drug treatments should be avoided if at all possible:
  - First-line: tricyclic anti-depressant e.g. amitripytline 25–75mg po
  nocte.
  - Second-line: short-term use of short-acting BDZ e.g. lorazepam
  0.5mg sublingually if difficulty initiating sleep and anxious.

Confusion

Definitions

- Confusion is a symptom of an organic brain syndrome.
- Chronic organic brain syndrome, or dementia, is a consequence of damage to cells within the brain and is irreversible.
- Acute organic brain syndrome, or delirium, is a consequence of physical illness. It can be reversible and involves global impairment of cognitive function:
  - Consciousness: less awake and alert.
  - Attention: poor concentration.
  - Perception: misinterpretation of sensory input.
  - Thinking: internal and external worlds confused.
  - Memory: new information cannot be stored.
  - Behaviour: agitated or withdrawn.

It is important to distinguish delirium from dementia (see Table 6.9). Patients with advanced respiratory disease are at risk of developing delirium. However, they are often elderly, and dementia may also be present.

Prevalence

- 5–40% of patients with advanced disease.
- 25–85% of patients in terminal phase (referred to as 'terminal agitation').

Consequences

- Highly negative impact on quality of life.
- Fear and distress (partial insight).
- Falls, fractures, and catheter/cannula withdrawal.
- Interference with control of other symptoms.
- Barrier to patient and family communication.
- Adverse effect on family grief.

Causes

Patients with advanced respiratory disease are at risk of developing delirium and consequent confusion for a number of reasons. Delirium is usually multi-factorial and many patients have a number of co-existing contributory factors:

- Drugs e.g. anticholinergic agents, steroids, benzodiazepines, opioids.
- Infection e.g. chest infection, urinary tract infection.
- Cerebral hypoxia e.g. respiratory failure, pulmonary embolism.
- Biochemical e.g. dehydration, hypercalcaemia, hyponatraemia.
- Others e.g. pain, severe anxiety, constipation.

Management

Assessment

- Undertake a detailed bedside clinical evaluation to determine whether confusion is a feature of delirium or dementia. Involve family/carers.
- Check that communication difficulties are not causing misdiagnosis, for example deafness or dysphasia.

- Limit investigations to those causes that are easily identified and effectively treated.
- Quantify severity of confusion using a mental test score (see Table 6.10 for an example).

Table 6.9 Features of delirium and dementia

Delirium	Dementia
• Acute	• Chronic
• Often reversible	• Irreversible
• Fluctuating	• Slowly progressive
• Clouding of consciousness	• Clear consciousness
• Information not taken in	• Information not retained
• Often aware and anxious	• Unaware and unconcerned
• Sleep disturbances	• Normal sleep amount
• Hallucinations	• Hallucinations rare
• Speech rambling and incoherent	• Speech stereotyped and limited
• Global cognitive impairment	• Memory changes apparent first

Table 6.10 Simplified mental test score

Question	Score
What is the date today? (day, month, year)	3
What is the address here? (three parts)	3
Can you take 7 away from 100? (93, 86, 79, 72, 65)	5
What is this called? (eg watch, pen, glass)	3
Remember and recall three imagined objects (after next task)	3
Three stage command (eg pick up paper in right hand, fold it, place it on table)	3
Total score	**20**

Correct potentially reversible causes
- Drugs
- Dehydration
- Infection
- Biochemical abnormalities
- Hypoxia

Non-pharmacological approaches
- Reduce fear and anxiety:
  - exploration and explanation
  - rationalization and reassurance
  - calm surroundings and familiar people.

- Orientate to reality:
  - well-lit environment
  - time cues e.g. clock, newspaper
  - regular daily schedule
  - use spectacles, hearing aids etc. as needed.

'Above all, the confused person needs constant reassurance by calm, sympathetic and familiar people, that he or she is safe, sane and understood.'

Kath Mannix

Pharmacological approaches
- Anti-psychotic medication:
  - Can lead to cognitive improvement, particularly of hallucinations, delusions, and paranoia.
  - Vary in sedative properties; haloperidol and risperidone are less sedating, levomepromazine and olanzapine are more sedating.
  - If drug treatment is required, haloperidol is recommended first-line (minimal anticholinergic and sedating effects and available through oral and parenteral routes).
- Benzodiazepines:
  - Can reduce anxiety and cause sedation.

- Use of sedating drugs will *not* reverse confusion and can often worsen it. A degree of sedation can further reduce a dwindling sense of reality and orientation. Avoid using sedative medications in confused patients other than in emergency situations, such as uncontrollable and dangerous behaviour.
- The key to control of confusion lies in correction of the underlying cause(s) and non-pharmacological approaches.

Anorexia and weight loss

Weight loss is common in advanced respiratory disease and involves loss of both fat and muscle. It is associated with:

- muscle weakness
- diaphragmatic dysfunction
- respiratory failure
- poor quality of life
- increased mortality.

Weight loss in both malignant and benign disease is caused by two main mechanisms:

- Reduced food intake (anorexia) due to a number of factors that can reduce appetite and cause difficulty eating, such as:
  - breathlessness
  - fatigue
  - social isolation.
- Increased production of pro-inflammatory cytokines such as TNF-α and IL1 that lead to a wide range of effects, including:
  - anorexia, because of production of anorectic agents such as corticotrophin-releasing factor
  - early satiety, because of delayed gastric emptying
  - wasting of muscle, because of impaired protein synthesis and proteolysis
  - fat loss, because of lipolysis and energy wasting.

Inadequate calorie intake (first mechanism) leads predominantly to fat loss. A hypercatabolic, chronic inflammatory state (second mechanism) leads to loss of muscle as well as fat, which has a particularly adverse effect on respiratory function.

Cachexia is diagnosed when the following criteria are present:[1]

- unintentional weight loss (≥5%)
- BMI:
  - less than 22 in those aged ≥65 years
  - less than 20 in those aged <65 years
- albumin <35g/L
- low fat
- evidence of cytokine excess e.g. elevated C-reactive protein.

Management

Non-pharmacological approaches

- Provide small, well-presented meals of patient's favourite food.
- Encourage 'little and often', particularly when experiencing fatigue or early satiety.
- Make sure that food can be prepared for and accessed by socially isolated patients if they are too breathless or fatigued to do it themselves.
- Encourage patients to get dressed, eat at a table, and ideally eat with others; eating is a social habit.
- Give general dietary advice including full-fat food and substitution of water-based drinks with milk-based drinks.

- Consider using nutritional supplements. Compliance can be increased by serving chilled with ice, adding extra full-fat milk or fruit juice (according to whether juice- or milk-based), making into a smoothie by adding fresh fruit and ice cream, making into a jelly, or freezing to make an ice lolly or ice cubes.
- Use appropriate non-drug measures to reduce contributing symptoms such as breathlessness and fatigue (see 📖 Chapter 5 pp. 68–74 and Chapter 6 pp. 112–114 respectively).
- In far advanced disease, avoid contributing to the pressure felt by patients to eat and the guilt/helplessness felt by families when patients do not eat. Explain that a full, balanced diet is unnecessary at this stage. Paradoxically, reducing the pressure on patients to eat can increase the pleasure gained from eating and even enhance intake.

Pharmacological approaches

Increasing oral intake alone is generally ineffective, because of the underlying catabolic, chronic inflammatory state. A number of drugs appear to reduce weight loss through an anti-inflammatory effect, decreasing pro-inflammatory cytokines:

- Progestogens:
  - Megesterol acetate 80–160mg daily, up to maximum of 800mg daily.
- Corticosteroids:
  - Dexamethasone 4mg daily.
  - Prednisolone 10–20mg daily.
- Omega-3 fatty acids:
  - Eicosapentanoic acid (EPA) 1.5–2g daily.

These drugs should only be used in the short term and when non-pharmacological approaches have been exhausted, because:

- The evidence to support their use is, as yet, limited and conflicting.
- Progestogens and corticosteroids can cause muscle catabolism. Much of the morbidity of cachexia comes from the muscle loss and the resulting negative impact on respiratory muscle strength. This may therefore be exacerbated by these drugs.
- Progestogens and corticosteroids have significant adverse effect profiles, including increased risk of venous thrombosis, hyperglycaemia, osteoporosis, and psychological disturbances.

Reference

1. Morley JE, Thomas DR, Wilson M-MG (2006) Cachexia: pathophysiology and clinical relevance. *Am J Clinical Nutrition*; 83: 735–743.

Constipation

Constipation is a common and neglected symptom in patients with advanced respiratory disease. It is experienced by 30–70% of patients, particularly those with malignant disease, and by 80–90% of those on opioids. It occurs in this patient group for a number of reasons:

- diminished food, fibre, and fluid intake
- drugs, such as opioids, anticholinergic agents, and diuretics
- poor mobility due to breathlessness and fatigue.

Immobility is a particularly important cause in this patient group. It results in slower intestinal transit and also hinders patients from getting to a toilet. The longer stool stays in the large bowel, the greater the resorption of fluid from it, and the firmer and less easy to expel it becomes.

Management

General measures

- Stop or reduce the dose of constipating drugs; tramadol and fentanyl are less constipating than morphine.
- Increase intake of fluid, particularly fruit juice, and fibre.
- Encourage mobility and manage symptoms that are hindering it.
- Improve access to a toilet or commode with good privacy.
- Avoid using a bedpan if at all possible.
- Raise the toilet seat.
- Install arm rails to facilitate independence and use of accessory respiratory muscles.
- Support feet on a footstool to help brace abdominal muscles.

Oral laxatives

- Surface-wetting agents have a stool-softening action by lowering stool surface tension, allowing water to percolate into its substance:
  • Docusate sodium 100mg bd, increasing to maximum of 500mg daily.
- Osmotic laxatives retain water in the intestinal tract and have a stool-softening effect by hydrating hardened faeces. The increased faecal volume, in turn, stimulates peristalsis, so these drugs have a stimulating as well as stool-softening action:
  • Lactulose syrup 15ml bd.
  • Macrogol e.g. Movicol® 1 sachet bd to tds, up to 8 in 24 hours.
- Stimulant laxatives act mainly on the submucosal and myenteric plexus of the large intestine to stimulate peristalsis. They tend to be most effective when combined with a stool-softening agent:
  • Bisacodyl 10–20mg po nocte, increasing up to tds.
  • Senna 15mg nocte, increasing to bd or tds.
  • Sodium picosulfate 5–10mg nocte, up to maximum of 30mg daily.
- Bulk-forming agents increase faecal mass and therefore stimulate peristalsis. These drugs are *not* recommended in this patient group because of the risk of worsening constipation in patients with inadequate fluid intake. They are particularly ineffective for opioid-induced constipation:
  • Ispaghula husk e.g. Fybogel® 1 sachet bd.

Rectal measures
- Suppositories take 30 minutes to dissolve after insertion:
  - Glycerin suppositories soften and lubricate faeces.
  - Bisacodyl suppositories have a stimulant action and must be in contact with the rectal mucosa to be effective.
- Enemas:
  - Osmotic standard enemas (118–128mL) contain phosphates.
  - Osmotic micro-enemas (5mL) contain sodium citrate, sodium lauryl sulphoacetate, glycerin, and sorbitol.
  - Arachis oil enema (130mL) is a lubricant (note: check for peanut allergy). It is instilled and left overnight before giving a further stimulant suppository or osmotic enema.

Recommendations in advanced respiratory disease:
- Always undertake general, non-drug measures to reduce constipation.
- A combination of a stool softener (e.g. docusate) and bowel stimulant (e.g. senna) is usually most effective.
- Avoid lactulose as it tends to cause flatulence and abdominal cramps and needs to be taken with a large fluid volume.
- For faecal impaction try either arachis oil enema followed by bisacodyl suppository, or high-dose Movicol® for 3 days.
- All patients commenced on strong opioids should also be started on oral laxatives (including a bowel stimulant).

Nausea and vomiting

- Nausea is more unpleasant than vomiting and is comparable to pain in terms of the distress it causes.
- Significant adverse consequences of nausea and vomiting include dehydration, anorexia, weight loss, anxiety, depression, and inability to prepare food and function socially.

Causes

- Respiratory disease:
  - benign CRD: cough, anxiety, pain, constipation
  - lung cancer: all the above and hypercalcaemia, hyponatraemia, hepatomegaly, raised intracranial pressure (ICP).
- Treatment:
  - drugs: opioids, antibiotics, TCA, SSRI, digoxin, ferrous sulphate, NSAIDs
  - chemotherapy, radiotherapy.
- Concurrent morbidity:
  - chest infection, UTI
  - peptic ulcer disease, dyspepsia
  - candidiasis
  - motion sickness.

Management

The most important step is to determine the underlying cause of the symptom through detailed symptom evaluation. This will then allow:
- reversible causes to be found and treated
- the mechanism of the symptom to be established and the most appropriate anti-emetic to be chosen.

Assessment

Take a detailed history of the nausea and vomiting, not unlike a detailed 'pain history'. This should include:
- separate evaluation of nausea (feeling of needing to vomit) and vomiting
- severity and timing of each symptom, including relief/persistence of nausea after vomiting
- frequency of vomiting, symptom triggers, and diurnal variation
- associated symptoms such as headache and abdominal distension
- volume and content of vomitus.

Two common clinical pictures are given in Table 6.11. The clinical features of the symptoms can help guide towards the likely cause of the symptom.

As always, a full history and examination must be conducted, including a review of the drug regimen. The clinical picture can be used to guide this; if, for example, a chemical cause is anticipated, then it becomes even more appropriate to check serum biochemistry and recent drug changes.

Table 6.11 Typical clinical pictures of nausea and vomiting

Chemical causes	Bowel related causes
• Severe persistent nausea	• Early satiety
• Vomiting may not relieve nausea for long	• Relatively little nausea and fully relieved by vomit
• Smaller volume vomitus or retching	• Larger volume vomitus
	• Undigested food or faeculent vomitus
	• Associated symptoms eg abdominal colic

Reversible causes
- Causes that may be reversible include emetogenic drugs, cough, anxiety, constipation, and severe pain.
- It is particularly important to try to control anxiety. Nausea and vomiting both cause and are caused by anxiety. The resulting 'vicious cycle' can be broken if anxiety is reduced.

Non-pharmacological management
- Avoid exposure to foods that may trigger nausea.
- Try small, frequent snacks rather than large meals.
- Measures to curb anxiety are vital, including a calm, reassuring environment and relaxation techniques.

Pharmacological management
See Table 6.12 for details of dose, mechanisms of action, and indications.
- First-line anti-emetics:
  - Metoclopramide—gastric stasis and functional bowel obstruction.
  - Cyclizine—raised intracranial pressure or motion induced.
  - Haloperidol—chemical causes such as drugs.
- Second-line anti-emetics:
  - Levomepromazine—multi-factorial aetiology, requiring sedation.
  - Dexamethasone—chemical causes, raised ICP due to brain metastases.
  - 5HT3 receptor antagonists such as granisetron—chemical causes.
- Principles of anti-emetic prescribing:
  - Start with a first-line drug selected according to the most likely cause of symptoms.
  - Re-evaluate regularly.
  - If the first selected drug is ineffective, either substitute another first-line anti-emetic or try a combination of first-line drugs such as cyclizine and haloperidol.
  - Never combine metoclopramide and cyclizine, as the latter blocks the prokinetic action of the former.
  - Always use the subcutaneous route even for nausea without vomiting, as nausea causes delayed gastric emptying.
  - If symptoms persist, consider substituting a second-line anti-emetic (or adding, in the case of dexamethasone).

Table 6.12 Anti-emetic drugs used in advanced disease

Drug	Indications	Mechanism of action	Dose	Comments
Metoclopramide	Functional bowel obstruction Gastric stasis Gastritis	Prokinetic: D_2 antagonist + $5HT_4$ agonist Prokinetic cholinergic nerves from myenteric plexus inhibited by dopamine and stimulated by 5HT	10mg tds po 30mg/24hrs CSCI	Effect blocked by anti-muscarinic drugs e.g. cyclizine
Cyclizine	Raised intracranial pressure Movement related N+V Mechanical bowel obstruction	Antihistaminic and anti-muscarinic Acts on vomiting centre	50mg tds po 100–150mg/24hrs CSCI	Can cause irritation at injection site Can be sedating
Haloperidol	Chemical causes of N+V including renal failure, drugs	Butyrophenone anti-psychotic D_2 antagonist Acts on chemoreceptor trigger zone	1.5mg on/bd po 3–5mg/24hrs CSCI	Combines well with cyclizine Useful in patients with anxiety, hallucinations, hiccups etc.
Levomepromazine	Multi-factorial N+V	Phenothiazine anti-psychotic Very broad spectrum: D_2, H_1, ACH_M, and $5HT_2$ antagonist	6–6.25mg od/bd po/sc 6.25–12.5mg/24hrs CSCI Acts for 12–24hrs (CSCI not necessarily needed)	Usually substituted rather than added Sedating Can be used to replace drug combinations May lower seizure threshold
Dexamethasone	Multiple causes	May reduce permeability of BBB to emetogenic substances	4–8mg od, po, or sc	Usually added to existing anti-emetic regimen Give in morning to avoid sleep disturbance
Granisetron	Chemical causes of N+V Situations of serotonin release	$5HT_3$ antagonist	1mg od or bd po or sc Dose (sc) lasts 24hrs and therefore CSCI not needed	Advantages over ondansetron: only once daily, and as effective po as sc Constipating

CSCI: continuous subcutaneous infusion; po: oral; sc: subcutaneously; od: once daily; bd: twice daily; tds: three times daily; on: once at night; BBB: blood-brain barrier

Emergencies in advanced respiratory disease

Introduction

In any patient with advanced respiratory disease, deterioration as a consequence of one of many acute medical emergencies can occur. Although most events will be completely unexpected, a proportion can be predicted. Unless the patient is very close to death, a failure to recognize and treat reversible symptomatology can cause distress and will increase patient morbidity.

In the event of any emergency in the palliative care setting, it is important to assess the following:

- Acute medical condition and burden of potential treatment.
- Wishes of the patient and family—implementation of a previously stated advance decision to refuse treatment (ADRT; previously known as a living will or advance directive) or care plan, recorded when the patient was mentally competent, will ensure patient autonomy is maintained during emergency situations. See Chapter 8 pp. 174–176.
- Prognosis of the patient's underlying disease—including an assessment of whether treatment will improve the quality of remaining life.
- Patient's recent performance status.

Planning ahead is of crucial importance. Anticipation of potential problems with preparation of the patient and care-giving team is vital to minimize patient discomfort and anxiety. Sensitive counselling about the risks of specific emergency events and potential limitations of available therapeutic options should be given. Emergency medications to minimize symptoms should be provided if appropriate, and arrangements should be made that take into account individual patients' pre-specified wishes, such as to remain at home.

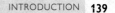

Acute pulmonary embolism

Acute pulmonary emboli (PE) are conventionally divided into massive (precipitating circulatory collapse) and non-massive types.

Clinical features

Massive PE
- Collapse with hypotension.
- Hypoxia.
- Acute right heart failure (e.g. elevated JVP).

Even a small pulmonary embolus can cause these catastrophic clinical sequelae in patients with limited respiratory reserve.

Non-massive PE
- Dyspnoea.
- Pleuritic chest pain.
- Cough.
- Haemoptysis.
- Tachypnoea.
- Tachycardia.
- Clinical DVT (approximately 10%).

Risk factors
- All patients with end-stage respiratory disease are at risk of pulmonary embolism.
- Malignancy and immobilization are both major risk factors (relative risk 5–20), and patients with COPD have a four-fold increased risk of PE as a consequence of associated immobility and related infections.

Diagnosis
- Assess pre-test clinical probability using a recognized scoring system e.g. British Thoracic Society (BTS, below), Wells, or Geneva scores.

British Thoracic Society Scoring System

A. Patient has clinical features compatible with PE:
tachypnoea ± haemoptysis ± pleuritic chest pain

Plus 2 other factors:
1. Absence of another reasonable clinical explanation.
2. Presence of a major risk factor.

A + 1 and 2: high pre-test clinical probability
A + 1 or 2: intermediate pre-test clinical probability
A alone: low pre-test clinical probability

Investigations

If clinical suspicion of PE is high, treatment should start prior to confirmatory investigations.

- D-dimer testing: perform depending on the pre-test probability score:
  - If low/intermediate pre-test score and negative d-dimer, PE can be excluded without further investigation.
  - If high pre-test score, further imaging required regardless of d-dimer.
  - The d-dimer level may be elevated as a result of the underlying disease and therefore its clinical applicability is often low.
- ECG: often sinus tachycardia or non-specific ST-T changes. S1Q3T3 is uncommon.
- CXR: may be normal. Occasionally reveals raised hemi-diaphragm, ipsilateral pleural effusion (~40%), segmental collapse, or wedge-shaped infarct. May detect other pathology.
- Arterial blood gas: increased alveolar to arterial (A-a) gradient i.e. VQ mismatch, ± hypoxia.
- CTPA: gold standard test (sensitivity >95%)—see Figure 7.1:
  - Many patients with underlying lung disease will have an abnormal chest radiograph and therefore CTPA is recommended as the first-line test for most patients with suspected PE.
- Ventilation/perfusion (V/Q) imaging: superseded by CTPA. Further investigation is required if indeterminate scan or discordant pre-test probability score and result.
- Doppler lower limb ultrasound: approximately 70% with PE have a proximal DVT so may be used as surrogate test in patients with clinical DVT.

Prognosis

- The mortality from an acute massive PE is ~20%.
- Haemodynamic instability as a consequence of acute right heart failure is associated with a worse prognosis.

Management

- 100% oxygen.
- Intravenous access, baseline bloods (FBC, clotting, liver, and renal function).
- Intravenous fluids to maintain right ventricular filling; if hypotension persists, inotropes should be considered.
- Anticoagulation:
  - IV unfractionated heparin (quicker onset of action) in massive PE or with renal failure.
  - Low molecular weight heparin (LMWH).
  - Consider oral anticoagulation once PE confirmed.

Note: use of oral anticoagulants in patients with advanced disease can be problematic. INR values can fluctuate for a variety of reasons (e.g. increased risk of drug interactions, liver impairment etc.). Patients require frequent blood checks and are at heightened risk of adverse effects. Daily subcutaneous LMWH offers a practical alternative with no need for monitoring of levels. In patients with cancer, randomized trial data also suggest that LMWH is more effective in reducing the risk of thromboembolism compared with oral anticoagulation; and it may have an additional anti-neoplastic effect.

- Thrombolysis, surgical embolectomy, and inferior vena caval filter insertion are all management options that are rarely used in patients with advanced, incurable disease.

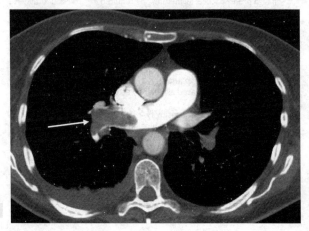

Fig. 7.1 Extensive thrombus extending from the main pulmonary artery and almost completely filling the right pulmonary artery (arrow).

Superior vena cava obstruction

Case history

A 60-year-old woman with recently diagnosed small cell lung cancer presented with worsening neck and facial swelling and progressive breathlessness. There was no cough, voice change, or syncope. On physical examination she had superficial venous distension and oedema over her chest wall and neck. Contrast-enhanced CT imaging showed almost total superior vena cava obstruction (SVCO) with multiple collateral pathways. She was started on dexamethasone 4mg qds and systemic chemotherapy was initiated. Symptomatic improvement was apparent within 7 days.

Introduction

SVCO results from obstruction of blood flow within the superior vena cava. It most commonly arises as a result of:

- Direct invasion or external compression of the vessel wall, usually by pathology to the right of the midline (80% of SVCO cases, as the SVC traverses the right side of the mediastinum into the right atrium), or by mediastinal structures e.g. lymph nodes.
- Less commonly SVCO is caused by intra-luminal thrombus.
- Occasionally these may co-exist.

Pathophysiology

A collateral venous network, particularly from the azygos vein, forms when the SVC is obstructed. Failure to establish a sufficient collateral circulation to accommodate the blood flow within the SVC, such as secondary to accelerated tumour growth, often results in rapid symptom development (over days to weeks) as a consequence of upper body oedema. Cerebral, nasal, and laryngeal oedema are rare.

Aetiology

Malignant causes

Malignancy is the most common cause of SVCO (60–85%) and should be considered in all patients.

- Lung cancer and lymphoma account for approximately 95% of all cases of malignant SVCO.
- Lung cancer is the most common cause of SVCO. 2–4% of all lung cancer patients and 10% of those with small cell lung cancer will develop SVCO at some point in their disease course.
- Lymphoma (almost invariably non-Hodgkin's lymphoma) causes SVCO in up to 4% of patients as a result of extrinsic lymph node compression. Hodgkin's lymphoma seldom causes SVCO.
- Thymoma, germ cell tumours, and metastatic mediastinal lymph node deposits (particularly breast) may also present with SVCO.

Benign causes

Non-malignant conditions account for approximately one-third of cases.

- SVCO secondary to SVC thrombosis is associated with use of indwelling central venous devices such as pacemakers and dialysis catheters.
- Fibrosing mediastinitis and infection, e.g. syphilitic thoracic aortic aneurysm and TB, are now rare causes.
- Radiation therapy, even if predating symptoms by several years, may induce local vascular fibrosis and precipitate SVCO.

Clinical features

- Dyspnoea.
- Facial and upper limb oedema, increased neck girth.
- Facial plethora with associated 'fullness' and headache, particularly on bending forward/lying down.
- Pemberton's sign (a constellation of facial plethora, distended head and neck superficial veins, and stridor upon raising the patient's arms above his/her head).
- Cough.
- Hoarseness.
- Stridor.
- Dysphagia.
- Cyanosis.
- Dizziness/pre-syncope/syncope.
- Confusion.
- Convulsions.
- Coma.

Diagnosis

SVCO is not usually immediately life-threatening and the diagnosis may be made clinically with radiological confirmation. Rarely, patients with SVCO can develop laryngeal oedema with stridor; such patients require emergency treatment as described below.

Investigations

Imaging

- CXR is abnormal in >80% of patients. It may show evidence of a lung primary, mediastinal widening, or pleural effusion.
- Contrast-enhanced CT of neck, chest, abdomen, and pelvis can suggest diagnosis and extent of underlying disease.
- MRI may be useful if contrast medium cannot be tolerated e.g. renal failure.

Tissue diagnosis

- CT may demonstrate a suitable biopsy site to obtain tissue for a histological diagnosis.
- Pre-biopsy radiotherapy may reduce the success rate of histology and corticosteroid use can make diagnosis of lymphoma difficult.
- Cytological diagnosis may be obtained from: pleural fluid (approximately two-thirds of patients with SVCO will have a pleural effusion), sputum, bronchoscopy, or lymph node aspiration. A core

biopsy sample rather than FNA is required for definitive lymphoma diagnosis.
- Although a tissue diagnosis is preferred to confirm malignant conditions and guide treatment, CT appearances may be sufficient to secure a diagnosis in very sick patients who are unfit for invasive investigations.

Management
- Treatment depends on the aetiology of the SVCO, and the severity of symptoms usually guides the urgency of treatment. Symptomatic improvement is usually seen within 1 to 2 weeks of treatment initiation.
- Outpatient management is often appropriate. However, emergency treatment is required for patients with laryngeal oedema and stridor.
- Patients with cancer and SVCO do not die of the syndrome itself but rather from the extent of their underlying disease. Survival amongst patients with malignancy-induced SVCO does not differ significantly from patients with a similar stage and type of tumour without SVCO.

General measures
- Elevate patient's head.
- Provide supplemental oxygen.
- Prescribe analgesia.
- Corticosteroids e.g. dexamethasone 8mg bd. Limited data to support their effectiveness but routinely used.

Specific treatment: malignant causes
- Treatment of underlying cause:
  - Palliative radiotherapy ± chemotherapy: initial treatment in NSCLC.
  - Chemotherapy alone: for chemo-sensitive tumours. Complete relief of symptoms is achieved in >80% of patients with SCLC or NHL and approximately 40% with NSCLC.
- Intravascular stent insertion can be considered in the following situations:
  - Severe symptoms prior to tissue diagnosis/radiotherapy.
  - Recurrent SVCO.
  - Patient not suitable for further oncological treatment.

Complications include infection, stent migration, pulmonary embolism, bleeding, and perforation. Low-dose anticoagulation (1mg warfarin aiming for INR <1.6) or aspirin is advocated by some centres for patients with SVC thrombus secondary to central venous devices. No definitive data exist to support this practice.

Specific treatment: benign causes
- Consider removal of intravascular devices.
- In patients with confirmed intravascular thrombus and who present within 5 days of symptom onset, thrombolysis may be performed.
- Subsequent anticoagulation may prevent thrombus extension/recurrence.

Specific treatment: laryngeal oedema
- Institute general measures as above.
- Ensure the airway is secure and administer supplemental oxygen.
- Referral for SVC stenting should be performed urgently. Although it is appropriate to start treatment with steroids, they take time to work and give no immediate benefit.

Pleural effusion

Mr H is an 88-year-old retired joiner who had noticed 2 months of progressive exertional dyspnoea such that he was having difficulty managing alone at home. A chest radiograph showed a moderate left-sided pleural effusion and a 1.5L pleural aspiration afforded symptomatic relief (see Figure 7.2). Pleural fluid cytology confirmed underlying mesothelioma. A week later his fluid re-accumulated with associated breathlessness and he was admitted to the ward. An intercostal chest tube was inserted and 3L of pleural fluid was drained. Talc pleurodesis was performed once drainage had ceased. 4 weeks later Mr H was able to manage his daily activities but his chest radiograph showed re-accumulation of a small left effusion. This was observed, as he was clinically stable. However, 3 weeks later he became more breathless and his X-ray confirmed recurrence of a large left pleural effusion. An indwelling pleural catheter was therefore discussed with Mr H and inserted with no complications. He was educated on its use and, with support from his district nurse, obtained symptom control and a good independent quality of life, draining approximately 500mL of pleural fluid from his catheter twice weekly.

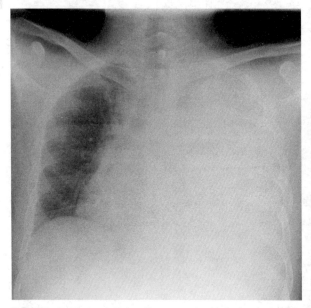

Fig. 7.2 Massive left pleural effusion with accompanying rightward mediastinal shift.

Introduction

- Pleural effusion is the presence of fluid in the pleural space, which occurs when there is an imbalance in the rate of physiological fluid production and absorption.
- There are over 55 documented causes of pleural effusion, which may be benign or malignant.
- Pleural effusion, particularly if recurrent, can result in significant patient morbidity.

Causes

- Benign:
  - Congestive cardiac failure and pneumonia are the commonest causes of pleural effusion in the Western world.
  - Other causes include pulmonary emboli, tuberculosis, and, less commonly, rheumatoid arthritis and other connective tissue diseases.
- Malignant:
  - Malignant pleural effusions are common and affect approximately 300,000 patients in the UK and US each year.
  - More than 75% of malignant pleural effusions (MPE) are caused by carcinoma of the lung, breast, ovary, mesothelioma, or lymphoma; they result from direct pleural involvement.
  - Para-neoplastic effusions result from indirect phenomena (e.g. bronchial obstruction, pulmonary embolism, or lymph node invasion).

Clinical features

- Breathlessness.
- Cough.
- Chest pain.
- Anorexia, weight loss.
- Malaise, fatigue.

Not all effusions cause symptoms, and an effusion may be an incidental finding in an asymptomatic patient.

Investigations

Diagnostic thoracentesis

If the cause of the effusion is unknown, a diagnostic thoracentesis (pleural aspiration) should be performed.

- Malignancy is the most common cause of an exudative pleural effusion in those >60yrs (around 5% of transudative effusions are malignant).
- Pleural fluid cytology sensitivity for malignancy is approximately 60% on the initial aspirate, increased slightly with analysis of a second sample.
- In patients with typical clinical features of heart failure, pleural aspiration is not required.

Imaging

- Chest X-ray with lateral view can give valuable information.
- Thoracic ultrasound may be needed to guide the site of pleural aspiration.
- Contrast-enhanced chest CT may distinguish benign from malignant disease.

Pleural tissue biopsy
- If the cause remains unclear, pleural tissue histology and culture may be indicated.
- Imaging-guided and thoracoscopic biopsies are superior to Abram's closed biopsies for detection of malignant disease.

Management

Key points influencing the treatment of pleural effusion include:
- Underlying cause.
- Patient symptoms, performance status, and wishes.
- If malignant: tumour sensitivity to, and patient suitability for, systemic therapy.
- Response to therapeutic thoracentesis.
- Patient prognosis.

Malignant pleural effusion
The median survival of patients with malignant pleural effusion is 4 months. Pleural interventions (see below) should only be performed if alleviation of symptoms is likely as a consequence, and invasive procedures should be minimized.
  Options include:
- Observation with close follow-up if asymptomatic.
- Therapeutic thoracentesis alone:
  - Removal of 1–1.5L affords symptom relief and allows assessment of the clinical response to fluid drainage.
  - Most malignant effusions will return within 30 days. However, one-off thoracentesis is appropriate in those with short predicted survival.
- Intercostal drainage and chemical pleurodesis via chest tube.
  - If symptoms are relieved following thoracentesis but then return with evidence of fluid recurrence, pleurodesis is generally recommended. This is the iatrogenic adhesion of the pleural surfaces to prevent pleural fluid accumulation.
  - Complete evacuation of the effusion via a small-bore chest drain precedes instillation of a sclerosing agent. Talc is the most commonly used sclerosant with a reported 71–96% success rate.
  - Chest pain, fever, dyspnoea, respiratory failure, and empyema are all recognized side effects of pleurodesis.
- Thoracoscopic pleurodesis:
  - Thoracoscopy allows diagnostic pleural biopsy and therapeutic pleurodesis during the same procedure. In those with known pleural malignancy, it offers little therapeutic advantage.
- Repeated therapeutic pleural aspirations:
  - If the lung does not fully re-expand following fluid removal ('trapped lung'), pleural apposition will not be achieved and pleurodesis will fail. In this situation, if symptoms related to pleural effusion presence persist, repeated therapeutic pleural aspiration may be required. This should be limited to those with a short life expectancy to reduce associated side effects such as pleural infection, patient discomfort, and pneumothorax. An indwelling pleural catheter is an alternative.

- Indwelling pleural catheter insertion:
  - This is indicated for patients with rapid re-accumulation of symptomatic pleural effusion, e.g. 'trapped lung'/failed pleurodesis, requiring frequent pleural aspiration.
  - The indwelling catheter allows outpatient control of pleural fluid and is associated with a spontaneous pleurodesis rate of up to 58%.
  - Risks include pleural infection and subcutaneous tumour spread along the catheter track.
- Pleuroperitoneal shunt:
  - A shunt may be used for patients with recurrent symptomatic effusions. Shunt occlusion (~10%) and infection are recognized complications.

Non-malignant pleural effusion
- Optimize conventional therapeutic measures for underlying condition.
- Use the above measures in patients who fail to respond.

In all patients, the non-pharmacological and pharmacological approaches to palliate breathlessness detailed in Chapter 5 should be used in tandem with the above measures, in order to optimize symptom control.

Airway obstruction

Introduction

- Primary or secondary thoracic tumours may be associated with airway obstruction (intrinsic, extrinsic, or both).
- The accompanying risk of post-obstructive collapse, infection, abscess formation, or haemoptysis can precipitate a sudden deterioration in a previously stable patient.
- Action to maintain airway patency reduces patient morbidity by recruitment of non-aerated lung and improvement of gas exchange.

Clinical features

- Increased dyspnoea.
- Sudden onset of respiratory distress, particularly in patients with known malignant tracheobronchial disease.
- Extreme agitation and distress, more commonly seen in patients with upper airway (tracheal) obstruction than in those with bronchial occlusion.
- Cyanosis.
- Respiratory distress.
- Imminent collapse with cardiorespiratory arrest.

Table 7.1 Clinical features of airway obstruction

Complete obstruction	Partial obstruction
Silent over collapsed lobe/lung	Noisy breathing/gurgling
Aphonia	Inspiratory stridor
Marked respiratory effort with tracheal tug/intercostal recession	Paradoxical thoraco-abdominal movement ('see-saw breathing')

Investigations

Intervention should precede investigations in the acutely distressed or peri-arrest patient.

- CXR and CT imaging may demonstrate lobar or complete lung collapse. Tomography also allows detailing of airway anatomy. Demonstration of a patent bronchus distal to the site of obstruction is essential to assess if endobronchial treatment is worthwhile. Other potentially confounding pathology e.g. pleural effusion and disease progression can be quantified.
- Flexible fibre-optic bronchoscopy allows assessment of the extent of the obstruction. Retained secretions that may be compounding the blockage can be removed.

Management

Airway obstruction is a frightening experience for patients and carers alike, and achieving symptom control is essential.

Acute management
- Acute upper airway obstruction:
  - Basic manoeuvres to obtain airway patency can be tried, such as a chin lift and/or jaw thrust, with suction of excess secretions and adjuvant airway devices. However, these are not usually successful if there is a mechanical occlusion and definitive treatment (see below) is often required.
  - Administration of Heliox (79% helium, 21% oxygen mixture) can alleviate symptoms of airway obstruction. Airway resistance is lowered with Heliox (due to its low density), thereby reducing 'work of breathing'.
  - Nebulized adrenaline (epinephrine) 1ml of 1:1000 diluted to a volume of 5mL with 0.9% saline can be used in patients who are not well enough for radiotherapy. It is thought to act through an α-adrenergic mediated vasoconstriction, which reduces laryngeal oedema.
  - See 📖 Chapter 5 for alternative measures for dyspnoea control.
- Malignant large airway obstruction:
  - Start dexamethasone 8mg bd.
  - Arrange urgent bronchoscopy ± CT imaging.
  - Consider palliative radiotherapy ± endobronchial intervention (see below).

Endobronchial techniques
These techniques are available only in specialist centres.

1. Airway stenting
Endobronchial lesions suitable for stenting are uncommon and careful patient selection is important.
- Consider in patients with inoperable underlying disease, with symptoms secondary to airway obstruction.
- Post-obstructive distal airway patency must be demonstrated.
- If attendant atelectasis has persisted for >2 weeks it is unlikely that significant re-expansion will be achieved.
- Stent insertion can be via rigid or flexible bronchoscopy (self-expandable stents).
- Patient mortality is unaffected; however, effective symptom palliation is seen in 80–90% of patients with tumour-related airway stenosis.
- Stent models may be custom-made, silicone or metallic, and covered or uncovered.
- Complications include malpositioning, airway wall perforation, and haemorrhage (procedural). Post-insertion complications include infection, stent migration, tumour in-growth (particularly with uncovered stents), secretion retention, and granulation tissue formation.
- Re-intervention or stent removal/exchange may be required.

2. Diathermy

3. Laser (Nd: YAG or CO_2) therapy

4. *Cryotherapy, brachytherapy (local radiotherapy) and photodynamic therapy*
- These have a delayed therapeutic effect and are inappropriate for patients with impending airway obstruction.

For patients where endobronchial therapy is not indicated or available:
- Optimize treatment of co-morbidities.
- Treat infection promptly.
- Use non-invasive measures for dyspnoea control (see 📖 Chapter 5).

Massive haemoptysis

- Haemoptysis, the expectoration of blood or blood-streaked sputum, is a common manifestation of underlying lung disease.
- Small-volume haemoptyses are usually self-limiting, and in approximately one-third of patients no cause will be found. They rarely herald a more significant bleed.
- Massive haemoptysis (>100mL fresh blood/24hrs) is less common, and can be potentially life-threatening as a result of asphyxiation. It carries a mortality rate of up to 80% and is distressing for patients, carers, and medical staff.

Aetiology

Table 7.2 Causes of massive haemoptysis

Common	Less common
Endobronchial malignancy	Lung abscess/mycetoma
Infection/TB	Diffuse alveolar haemorrhage/ vasculitides
Bronchiectasis	
Pulmonary embolism	Cardiovascular – AV malformations, mitral stenosis, pulmonary hypertension, aortic aneurysm
Bleeding diathesis/anticoagulation	
Iatrogenic (e.g. post bronchoscopy)	Pulmonary haemosiderosis
	Invasive aspergillosis

Management

- Massive haemoptysis is a medical emergency.
- Approach calmly as patients are inevitably very frightened.
- Active intervention is not appropriate for all patients and treatment should be instituted on an individual patient basis.

Acute management

- Manage in an appropriate setting, if possible, such as HDU/ITU.
- Ensure airway protection:
  - Arrange endotracheal intubation if poor gas exchange, ongoing haemoptysis, or haemodynamic instability.
  - Apply high-flow supplemental oxygen if intubation is not required.
- Cardiovascular support:
  - 2× large-bore IV access.
  - Intravenous fluid resuscitation.
  - Reverse any bleeding diathesis.
  - Consider inotropes.
- Nebulized adrenaline (5–10mL of 1:10,000).
- Protect non-bleeding lung if location of bleed is known (e.g. post bronchoscopic biopsy):
  - Lie patient in lateral position with the bleeding lung downward. This prevents spillage into the 'clean' lung.

- In intubated patients, placement of a single-lumen endotracheal tube into the non-bleeding lung, or placement of a double-lumen ET tube, may be considered.
- Bronchoscopy:
  - Fibre-optic bronchoscopy seldom has a role in an acute massive bleed.
  - Rigid bronchoscopy (under general anaesthetic) can allow identification of bleeding site and haemostasis (e.g. topical adrenaline, iced-saline lavage, laser therapy, electrocautery).
- If bleeding continues consider the following:
  - Bronchial arteriography and embolization—requires active bleeding at the time of investigation to identify the leaking vessel (50% of patients have recurrent bleeds).
  - Surgery—usually a last resort e.g. segmentectomy, lobectomy, or pneumonectomy.

Other measures
- Antifibrinolytic agents such as tranexamic acid (0.5–1g tds orally or IV) stabilize clot formation by inhibition of tissue fibrinolysis, and may be successful in preventing excessive bleeding.
- Treat concomitant infection with antibiotics.
- Correct coagulation defects.
- Consider external beam radiotherapy (or laser therapy) directed at the bleeding site.

In patients with a poor prognosis, aggressive intervention may be inappropriate and relief of symptoms is of paramount importance:
- Analgesia and sedation (with parenteral opiates or benzodiazepines), cough suppression, supplemental oxygen, and regular oropharyngeal suction may be useful.
- If haemoptysis continues, selective use of the above measures may still be appropriate to achieve symptom palliation.

Secondary spontaneous pneumothorax

Definition

- A secondary spontaneous pneumothorax is the presence of air in the pleural space of patients *with underlying lung disease* (in comparison to spontaneous primary pneumothoraces, which occur in people with apparently normal lungs).
- Patients with COPD account for 60% of secondary pneumothoraces. Other associated conditions include interstitial lung disease (see Figure 7.3), asthma, lung cancer, *Pneumocystis jiroveci* infection (pneumocystis carinii pneumonia, PCP), and cystic fibrosis.
- Smoking is a major risk factor.

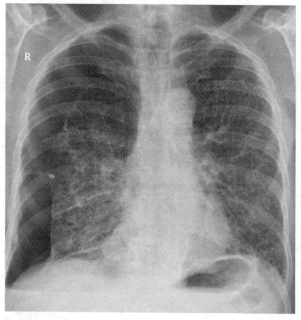

Fig. 7.3 Large right secondary pneumothorax in 72-year-old man with interstitial lung disease; note the presence of an intercostal chest drain.

Clinical features

- Patients commonly develop pleuritic chest pain and/or breathlessness.
- Even a small pneumothorax can create dyspnoea, which seems out of proportion to its size in patients with little underlying respiratory reserve.
- There is typically ipsilateral reduced expansion, hyper-resonance, and diminished air entry. These signs may be difficult to elicit in those with chronic obstructive airways disease and lung hyperinflation.

Investigations

- Chest X-ray:
  - Look for absence of lung markings with a visible lung edge and features of the underlying lung disease.
  - A rim of air >2cm defines a large pneumothorax (approximately 50% volume).
- Thoracic CT may be needed to differentiate secondary pneumothorax from underlying bullous lung disease.

Management

Secondary spontaneous pneumothorax has a mortality of 10% and a recurrence rate of approximately 45%.

Treatment aims to (1) remove air from the pleural space to afford relief of symptoms, and (2) reduce recurrence risk and adherent morbidity.

- Specialist advice should be sought.
- In all patients, apply oxygen (controlled FiO_2 if indicated) and optimize treatment of the underlying condition.
- Intercostal tube drainage is the first-line treatment in most cases (see box below).
- Pleural aspiration is only indicated if the patient is asymptomatic and has a small (<2cm rim) pneumothorax.
- A persistent air leak occurs (i.e. the chest drain continues to bubble) in approximately one in five patients with a secondary spontaneous pneumothorax, particularly in the elderly. Application of chest tube suction (-5 to -20cm H_2O) should be considered.
- When the lung re-expands, chemical pleurodesis (i.e. with talc slurry) via the chest tube should be performed to reduce the risk of recurrence.
- If the lung remains unexpanded or there is an air leak persisting after 5–7 days, surgical treatment (video-assisted thoracoscopic surgery (VATS) or open thoracotomy) can be considered. Several studies have demonstrated efficacy in elderly patients and those with poor prior lung function. However, selection criteria for surgery vary between units. Factors that often preclude operative intervention are hypercapnia ($PaCO_2$ >7kPa), poor previous exercise tolerance (<150 yards), and associated cardiovascular disease. Mechanical (pleural abrasion) or chemical (talc poudrage) pleurodesis is performed during surgery.
- In patients not suitable, or keen, for surgery, chemical pleurodesis via the chest tube can be attempted. An alternative, which allows outpatient management, is the insertion of a Heimlich one-way flutter valve.

Practical point: Seldinger chest drain insertion[1]

Important note: Chest drain insertion is associated with significant potential morbidity and mortality. Image guidance, e.g. ultrasound or CT, should be used whenever available and only an experienced operator should perform the procedure. All patients who have a chest drain placed should be looked after on a ward with staff who are experienced and competent in their management.

- Confirm indication for drain insertion.
- Ensure you have all the necessary equipment including chest drain bottle and tubing.
- Obtain written and verbal consent from patient.
- Administer pre-medication e.g. midazolam 1–5mg intravenously and/or opiates IV/SC/orally if required.
- Position the patient appropriately. For most large pneumothoraces the patient should lie at 45° with their ipsilateral arm raised behind their head. (Patients could also be positioned in the left or right lateral position or sitting forward resting their arms over a table—the latter posterolateral approach is safe but patients are subsequently unable to lie back comfortably.)
- Aim to insert the drain in the mid-axillary line, 4th or 5th intercostal space within the 'triangle of safety'—demarcated anteriorly by lateral border of pectoralis major, posteriorly by the posterior axillary line, and inferiorly by a line drawn laterally from the nipple.
- Using a sterile technique, prepare all equipment and sterilize the hemithorax using a chlorhexidine or an iodine-based wash.
- Infiltrate with lidocaine local anaesthetic (10–20mL of 1 or 2%) until you reach the pleural surface and freely aspirate air (or fluid).
- Open the Seldinger drain kit.
- Make a small skin incision (~5mm) parallel to the upper surface of the underlying (usually 4th or 5th) rib, using the scalpel provided.
- Insert the introducer needle and once you are able to aspirate air/fluid, remove the syringe and feed the guidewire into the pleural cavity through the needle. One hand should always be in contact with the guidewire.
- Remove the needle leaving the wire in place.
- Dilate the tract to the pleural surface by inserting the dilator over the wire—you do not need to insert this more than 2cm once you feel it enter the pleural space.
- Remove the dilator and insert the drain over the wire (10–14cm is sufficient).
- Remove the guidewire and attach three-way tap.
- Insert a holding suture (one method is to place a loose stitch ~5–10mm adjacent to the drain insertion site and then tie individual loops from this around the tube) and secure with an adhesive dressing.
- Connect the drain tubing and bottle.
- Ensure the drain is bubbling (or draining) appropriately.
- Give the patient clear (written if available) instructions on drain care.
- Request a check radiograph to assess drain positioning and underlying lung.

Reference

1. Havelock T, Teoh R, Laws D, Gleeson F. Pleural procedures and thoracic ultrasound: British Thoracic Society pleural disease guideline. *Thorax* 2010, 65 (suppl II) ii 61–ii 76.

Hypercalcaemia

Definition

Hypercalcaemia occurs when corrected serum calcium levels exceed 2.60mmol/L. However, symptoms are unusual unless levels are >3.0mmol/L. Severe hypercalcaemia (>3.5mmol/L) needs prompt treatment.

Aetiology

- 10–20% of patients with cancer develop hypercalcaemia (40% with myeloma).
- In lung cancer, hypercalcaemia may arise through various mechanisms. It may be precipitated by ectopic parathyroid hormone-related peptide (PTHrP) secretion or the release of local cytokine mediators e.g. transforming growth factor-alpha (TGF-α), interleukin-1 (IL1), or tumour necrosis factor-alpha and -beta (TNF-α/β). Less frequently, increased osteoclastic bone activity as a consequence of skeletal metastases can result in hypercalcaemia.
- Incidental primary hyperparathyroidism can occur rarely.

Clinical features

Clinicians need to remain vigilant as symptoms are often non-specific and may mimic the underlying disease.

The phrase 'bones, stones, abdominal groans, and psychic moans' describes the classic constellation of symptoms:
- Abdominal pain.
- Vomiting.
- Nausea.
- Anorexia.
- Constipation.
- Weight loss.
- Fatigue, weakness.
- Confusion.
- Cardiac arrhythmias.
- Pancreatitis.
- Renal stones, renal failure.

Investigations

- Serum biochemistry:
  - Bone profile: alkaline phosphatase, phosphate (low in hyperparathyroidism and ectopic PTHrP), and albumin (often low in malignancy).
  - Electrolytes, urea, creatinine.
- Serum PTH levels: should be suppressed; high levels suggest hyperparathyroidism.
- Imaging: isotope bone scanning/MRI may identify metastatic bony deposits.
- ECG: short Q-T interval, lengthened T-wave duration.

Management

- Rehydration:
  - This alone can reduce corrected calcium levels by 0.2–0.4mmol/L.
  - Use 0.9% saline.
  - Supplement with K^+ if hypokalaemic.
  - Avoid fluid overload and aim for 4–6L in 24 hours.
- Bisphosphonates:
  - Use in hypercalcaemia of malignancy.
  - Act by reducing osteoclast action and hence bony resorption.
  - Options include disodium pamidronate (30–90mg in 500mL 5% glucose or sodium chloride 0.9% over 2 hours) or zoledronic acid (4mg in 100mL 5% glucose or sodium chloride 0.9% over at least 15 minutes).
  - Maximal effect is at 1 week.
- Corticosteroids:
  - Examples include prednisolone 30–60mg daily or dexamethasone 6–12mg daily.
  - May help by reducing intestinal absorption and increasing urinary excretion.
  - Are more valuable in myeloma, sarcoidosis-related hypercalcaemia, and vitamin D excess.
- Diuretics e.g. furosemide 40mg bd (po/IV):
  - Use once adequately hydrated to encourage renal calcium excretion.
- Salmon calcitonin (8U/kg/8h IM):
  - Can use in resistant hypercalcaemia.
  - Acts through inhibition of bone reabsorption and an increase in calcium excretion.
  - However, its duration of action is short and alternative agents (as above) are favoured.
- Other measures include:
  - Use haloperidol for relief of nausea and vomiting (effective for chemical causes of nausea because of action on central D2 receptors in the chemoreceptor trigger zone).
  - Stop contributory medication, such as thiazide diuretics.

Prognosis

Hypercalcaemia of malignancy is a poor prognostic sign with a median 1-year survival of approximately 20%. Untreated median survival is less than 1 month.

Syndrome of inappropriate ADH secretion

Definition
The excessive retention of water due to 'inappropriate' continued secretion of antidiuretic hormone (ADH, vasopressin) despite plasma hypotonicity.

Aetiology
- Malignancy:
  - e.g. lung, particularly SCLC (ectopic secretion of ADH), mesothelioma, lymphoma, gastrointestinal, genitourinary tract.
- Chest disease:
  - eg. bronchopneumonia, tuberculosis.
- Central nervous system disorders:
  - eg. infection, stroke, head injury.
- Drugs:
  - e.g. opioids, chlorpropramide, SSRIs, tricyclic anti-depressants, carbamazepine.
- Metabolic disease:
  - e.g. alcohol withdrawal, porphyria.

Clinical features
- Depend on severity and rate of change of serum sodium.
- Include nausea, lethargy, irritability, headache, and anorexia if <125mmol/L.
- Severe hyponatraemia (<120mmol/L) may result in confusion, seizures, or coma.

Investigations/Diagnosis
Diagnosis requires presence of:
- Hyponatraemia (<125mmol/L).
- Low plasma osmolality (<260mOsm/kg).
- Concentrated urine (sodium >20mmol/L, usually >40mmol/L).
- Urinary osmolality >100mOsm/kg.
- Clinical euvolaemia with no evidence of hypovolaemia/oedema.
- No recent use of diuretics.
- Normal thyroid, renal, and adrenal function.

Management
- Treat the cause.
- Restrict fluid intake: 0.5–1L/24hrs.
- Consider demeclocycline 300–600mg bd (inhibits ADH activity at the distal renal tubule).
- Encourage dietary salt and protein intake.
- Vasopressin-receptor (V_{1A} and V_2) antagonist therapy (conivaptan) has recently been approved for intravenous use in euvolaemic hyponatraemia and may be considered if available. Oral vasopressin-receptor (V_2) antagonists are not yet clinically available.

In emergency cases (seizures, coma):
- Consider infusion of normal (0.9%) or hypertonic saline (1.8% or 3%) at 1–2mL/kg of body weight/hr.
- Concomitant furosemide can be given.
- Aim for a gradual increase in serum sodium to 125mmol/L as osmotic demyelination (central pontine and extrapontine myelinolysis) may be provoked with rapid correction.

Chapter 8

Communication with patients and families

Introduction

Inadequate communication is one of the greatest barriers to the provision of good end of life care. A number of studies have attempted to define a 'good death' (Table 8.1) and, unerringly, the majority of constructs rely on good communication between patients and healthcare professionals.

There are two vital components of high quality communication during end of life care:

- Acknowledgement of poor prognosis:
  - It is impossible to plan and receive good end of life care without communication that openly acknowledges progressive and irreversible disease with a limited prognosis.
- Advance care planning (ACP):
  - This is a process of discussion about future care that occurs between a patient and their healthcare provider. If the patient wishes, it may also include family or friends.
  - An ACP discussion may include the individual's concerns, preferred future place/providers of care, and future treatment preferences.

There is consistent evidence that the majority of patients (>70%) want to undertake these conversations. Patients with non-malignant chronic respiratory disease appear to have even greater information needs than those with cancer.[1,2] However, these needs are not being met.

- Many patients, particularly those with non-malignant disease, are never given the opportunity to take part in discussions about their prognosis, and their future wishes and preferences.
- There is research evidence that patients rate professionals poorly in the areas of discussion of prognosis and the process of dying.
- A large proportion of complaints about healthcare in acute hospitals relate to care at the end of life, and the majority of these reflect inadequate communication.

Early and good-quality communication is particularly important in advanced respiratory disease because of the typically unpredictable and rapid terminal decline. During an acute deterioration, there may be insufficient time to make plans and, furthermore, patients may lack capacity to make decisions regarding their future care. Healthcare professionals are notoriously poor in judging patients' quality of life and likely wishes and preferences. It is therefore vital that patients' views are clarified in advance.

Poor communication has a number of adverse consequences:

- Patients lose control, autonomy, and independence, the three factors most valued at the end of life.
- Fears and concerns are compounded by not being shared and addressed.
- Patients and carers lack time to make important preparations for death, such as organizing affairs, writing a will, and planning the funeral.
- Death may not occur in the place of choice and the people of choice may not be present.
- Unwanted life-prolonging measures may be continued inappropriately.

Table 8.1 Components of a 'good death'[3]

Clear decision making	Clear communication about treatment decisions and future wishes empowers patients.
Preparation for death	Patients and carers want to know what to expect, and to have time to prepare.
Completion	This may include life review, resolution of conflicts and saying goodbye.
Contributing to others	Patients may want to contribute to the well-being of others.
Affirmation of the whole person	This provides dignity, and respects the context of patients' lives, values and preferences.
Pain and symptom management	Control of symptoms can optimise comfort and quality of life

References

1. Curtis J, Wenrich M, Carline J, et al. (2002) Patients' perspectives on physician skill in end-of-life care: differences between patients with COPD, cancer, and AIDS. *Chest;* 122: 356–362.
2. Edmonds P, Karlsen S, Khan S, et al. (2001) A comparison of the palliative care needs of patients dying from chronic respiratory diseases and lung cancer. *Palliat Med;* 15: 287–295.
3 Steinhauser K, Clipp E, McNeilly M, et al. (2000) In search of a good death: observations of patients, families, and providers. *Ann Int Med* 132(10): 825–832.

Barriers to communication in advanced disease

There is strong evidence that the majority of patients with advanced respiratory disease wish to take part in advance care planning discussions, and yet only a minority are given this opportunity. A number of healthcare professional and patient factors hinder communication in those suffering from advanced respiratory disease.

Clinicians communicate badly for a number of reasons:
• Difficulty in timing discussions because of uncertain prognosis.
• Belief that patients are not ready to discuss end of life issues.
• Concern that frank communication will take away patients' hope.
• Fear that admission of poor prognosis would erode patients' and families' trust in medical staff.
• Reluctance to have to admit to 'failure' of medical treatment.
• Perceived lack of time in consultations.
• Lack of training in communication skills, particularly in relation to 'difficult conversations' about dying.
• Perceived conflict between the goals of chronic disease management, such as active self-management, and end of life care.

Patients, too, can hinder good quality communication because of a number of factors:
• An expectation that healthcare professionals will initiate discussions.
• Lack of understanding that non-malignant diseases, such as COPD, are life-limiting conditions.
• Uncertainty as to which clinicians will be involved during the end of life phase.
• Fear that discussion of dying would embarrass medical staff by implying treatment failure.
• Lack of certainty about the type of care that would be wanted when less well.
• Fear that staff will 'give up' on them earlier if they seem to have accepted that they are seriously ill.
• Societal taboos that inhibit open discussion of death and dying.

Uncertain prognosis

'Uncertainty is the only certainty there is, and knowing how to live with insecurity is the only security.'

John Allen Paulos

Accurate prognostication is virtually impossible in advanced non-malignant respiratory disease. This is the greatest impediment to good advance care planning. The typical illness trajectory involves a very slow decline, punctuated by brief episodes of acute deterioration, with death occurring unpredictably during any one such episode. The lack of a clear end of life phase makes timing advance care planning discussions difficult.
• Patients and their carers need information much earlier than is perceived by healthcare professionals.

- With sensitive communication, it is unlikely that discussions will occur too early.
- Timing difficulties should not lead to communication paralysis.

Societal taboos

Death and dying appears to be the last great taboo in the society of developed nations. Reduced mortality in younger people and the fact that most people now die in institutions has markedly reduced familiarity with dying. This leads to a societal lack of openness and discussion about death and dying, and hinders communication within families and between patients and professionals.

- This important deterrent to communication is increasingly being recognized, including at a national level. In the UK, the Dying Matters Coalition (see 📖 p. 191) has been set up to promote increased public awareness of death and dying.
- Schools, universities, religious organizations, solicitors, funeral directors, and hospices all have a role to play in promoting open discussion, contributing eventually to a shift in societal attitudes towards death. Some commentators have advocated a 'public health' approach, aiming to integrate and normalize end of life care within society.[1]

Fear of destroying hope

Healthcare professionals fear destroying patients' hope and become concerned that open discussion of a poor prognosis would be perceived as medical failure, eroding patients' trust in them. Although understandable, these concerns are unfounded, and indeed the converse may be true.

- Fears that are not discussed are often worse than reality.
- Hope and trust are sustained by open communication that both acknowledges reality and encourages development of realistic goals.
- Relationships between patients and clinicians are enhanced by compassionate communication that gives patients control, empowering them to plan for the future.

Reference

1. Kellehear A (2005) *Compassionate Cities: Public Health and End of Life Care.* Routledge, New York.

Discussion of prognosis

'Earlier recognition of people nearing the end of their life leads to earlier planning and better care.'

Gold Standards Framework

Communication about end of life care cannot, by definition, occur without acknowledgement of irreversible, progressive disease and a limited prognosis. Prediction of prognosis is, however, very difficult in those with advanced respiratory disease, particularly for those with chronic non-malignant lung disease. This difficulty forms the greatest impediment to discussion of prognosis and subsequent advance care planning.

Prediction of prognosis

Prognostication is considered in detail in 📖 Chapter 4, pp. 52–54. The unpredictable disease trajectory in advanced non-malignant disease makes prediction of prognosis particularly challenging.

Prognosticating in lung cancer

- Ask the 'surprise question', an intuitive question that integrates a large number of clinical factors: 'Would I be surprised if this patient were to die in the next 6–12 months?' If the answer is 'no', it is time to consider discussing prognosis and advance care planning.
- Assess the rate at which the patient's condition is changing. If deterioration occurs month by month, the prognosis may be measured in months; if week by week, in weeks; and if day by day, in days.
- Assess performance status. Patients that spend more than 50% of their waking time lying down tend to have a prognosis of less than 3 months.

Prognosticating in non-malignant chronic respiratory disease

Several prognostic models have been developed in patients with non-malignant disease that attempt to quantify an estimate of survival, such as the BODE index for patients with COPD (see 📖 Chapter 4, p. 53). Such formal scores tend to be unreliable because of the inherently unpredictable nature of the disease. Falsely positive predictions of survival can give an excuse to delay advance care planning discussions.

- Again, ask the 'surprise question': 'Would I be surprised if this patient were to die in the next 6–12 months?' On admission to hospital, always ask, 'Would I be surprised if this patient were to die during this admission?' If the answer is 'no', acknowledgement of prognosis and advance care planning is needed.
- Ask about severity of breathlessness. The degree of dyspnoea has been shown to be a more reliable indicator of both a poor prognosis and a willingness to discuss end of life issues than disease severity or pulmonary function.

Recommendation in advanced respiratory disease
Simple and intuitive triggers for the initiation of discussions of prognosis and advance care planning, such as the 'surprise question', are recommended above formal prediction scores.
- This pragmatic approach is easy, rapid, and feasible in patients with advanced disease.
- The intention is to anticipate the possibility of entering the last year of life and to trigger appropriate discussion, rather than to make a formal prediction of survival time.

Communicating prognosis

Good communication skills are a prerequisite for these sensitive discussions.
- Use open questions such as 'Have you any concerns about the future?' and 'What are you hoping that we might be able to achieve?'
- Pick up on cues from patients and carers, such as 'I'm worried that I'm not able to…' Expressions of 'worry' or anxiety reflect underlying concerns about the future.
- Respond to cues by showing willingness to talk about the future, and consider checking with the patient that this is what they would like to do. 'I can see that you're thinking about the future—I am too. Is this something you would like to talk about in a bit more detail?' Patients usually respond in the affirmative, and permission for further discussion has now been given.
- Encourage patients to undertake such discussions. 'Many people with advanced disease find that the fears in their mind are actually worse than the reality.' 'Sometimes talking about your worries can make them seem more manageable.'
- If there are no cues from the patient, broach the subject honestly and with compassion: 'We're not very good at predicting what the future holds with COPD. Sometimes people can live for several years with advanced disease, but if there is a sudden deterioration it is possible one can die much sooner.'
- 'Chunk and check': give small amounts of information at a time and check that the patient understands and wants to continue the discussion. Patients usually want to have these discussions but do need to feel in control of the content and extent of the conversation. Use the techniques for breaking bad news given on 📖 pp. 184–186.

Prognosticating is a notoriously inaccurate process. Both over- and underestimating prognosis can cause significant distress to both patients and their families. Talking in terms of 'many months', 'weeks to short months', 'days to short weeks' can be helpful, without being too specific.

Advance care planning

Definitions

Advance care planning (ACP) is a process of discussion about future care between a patient and their health carers. If the individual wishes, family and friends may be included in the discussion. Awareness of the life-limiting nature of the disease is a prerequisite to advance care planning. An ACP discussion may include:

• further exploration of understanding of the illness and prognosis
• eliciting the patient's concerns and fears
• discovering important values or personal goals of care
• establishing the patient's preferred place and providers of care
• discovering the patient's wishes for future treatment, such as antibiotics, NIV, or invasive ventilation.

Advance care planning differs from planning in general in that ACP takes place in the context of anticipated future deterioration, which may be associated with a loss of capacity to make decisions.

Principles

• The process of ACP is voluntary. Although most patients benefit from ACP discussions, some individuals do not wish to confront future issues, and this should be respected. Initiation of such discussion must always be undertaken sensitively.
• ACP should be a patient-centred dialogue, focusing on the views of the individual patient. It may be informed by the views of family members or friends that the patient invites to participate.
• ACP is a dynamic process; it usually entails a number of discussions over time. The discussions may also evolve, with changes in goals of care, concerns, and preferences.
• All staff involved in the care of patients with advanced disease should be alert to cues that an individual may wish to discuss the future.
• Staff initiating ACP discussions should be trained or competent in effective communication skills. They should have sufficient knowledge of treatment and care options to enable the patient to make an informed decision.
• Patient confidentiality should be respected, as always. Information should not be shared with family members or friends without the patient's consent. Sharing information with healthcare professionals should be on a 'need to know' basis.

Practical points

Timing

Patients usually expect healthcare professionals to initiate ACP discussions. A number of factors may provide a trigger for staff to consider advance care planning:

• A healthcare professional would not be surprised if the patient were to die within the next year (the 'surprise question', see 📖 p. 172).
• The patient gives cues that he/she is worrying about the future, for example by expressing concern about who will care for them at home.
• There have been multiple recent hospital admissions.

- Non-invasive ventilation has just been used for the first time during an acute exacerbation of disease.
- There has been a recent significant event such as the death of a spouse or close friend.

Setting

ACP discussions need to take place in a setting that is conducive to open and sensitive communication. Discussion should take place in a private, quiet, and comfortable room, with the prospect of 30 minutes or more of uninterrupted time. A busy hospital or general practice clinic setting, with 10-minute appointments, is rarely appropriate for advance care planning discussions. A number of settings can support fruitful ACP discussions:

- At home, for example a domiciliary visit by a specialist nurse.
- In a private room on a hospital ward, a day or so prior to discharge.
- In a hospice or respite care setting.

Capacity

A patient's capacity to decision-make should always be established prior to undertaking an ACP discussion. Capacity is decision-specific, so lack of capacity to make a particularly complex decision should not preclude all care planning discussions (see 📖 Chapter 9, pp. 198–199.)

Communication skills

Appropriate communication skills are a prerequisite to ACP discussions, and are described on 📖 pp. 178–186. Most professionals working with patients with advanced disease already have the ability to undertake care planning. A lack of confidence in using existing skills is more common than an actual lack of skill.

Documentation

It is vital to document accurately the outcome of any ACP discussion. This usually occurs in the form of a statement of preferences and wishes or, on occasion, a formal advance decision to refuse treatment (ADRT). Communication of the outcomes of the discussion to the healthcare teams involved in that patient's care across all settings is vital.

Statement of wishes and preferences

A statement summarizing beliefs, values, wishes, and preferences should be written in a patient's notes. This information should ideally also be written in a letter and sent to all other relevant health carers, as well as to the patient. The patient's confidentiality should be respected and consent for the information to be shared should be sought explicitly.

A statement of wishes and preferences is not legally binding, but does have legal standing. It must be taken into account and used to help judge 'best interest' for patients who lack the capacity to make decisions for themselves.

Advance decision to refuse treatment (ADRT)
A small minority of ACP discussions lead to the creation of a legally binding ADRT (see 📖 Chapter 9, p. 202). However, ADRTs are only of limited use. Future medical events can usually not be predicted in detail, and the advance decision may no longer be valid or applicable at the time when it is needed. Overall the drive and focus of ACP should be on establishing a patient's wishes and preferences, rather than on the creation of a legally binding document.

Key points:
- Advance care planning (ACP) should occur when a person is slowly deteriorating, rather than during an acute exacerbation.
- ACP should occur early in case of future loss of capacity. It is not 'someone else's problem'; take responsibility and organize promptly.
- Patients expect healthcare professionals to initiate the discussion.
- Choose the timing and context carefully whenever possible, but do not use logistical difficulties as an excuse for failing to initiate ACP.
- Most patients wish to undertake ACP discussions; the minority who do not should not be pressured to agree to discussion.
- ACP is a dynamic process that is rarely completed during a single discussion.
- An open question style of dialogue is key to successful ACP.
- Initiation of treatments that may be difficult to withdraw, such as NIV, should be preceded by ACP discussions.
- The outcomes of an ACP discussion should be documented in a statement of wishes and preferences.

Practical communication skills

'When people talk, listen completely. Most people never listen.'
Ernest Hemingway

Good communication is a basic clinical skill. There is evidence that effective communication skills can lead to a wide range of benefits:
- Patients' problems and concerns are identified more accurately, and health outcomes improve as a result.
- Patient satisfaction increases significantly. Psychological distress reduces and patients adjust more quickly to challenging circumstances.
- Patient compliance improves, and they become more likely to adhere to treatment or advice given.
- Clinicians with good communication skills experience greater job satisfaction and less work stress.

Challenges in respiratory disease

Communicating with patients with advanced respiratory disease can be particularly challenging. A number of factors mean that professionals working with patients with advanced respiratory disease need to have particularly effective communication skills:
- Deterioration in condition can occur very rapidly, giving limited time for communication and establishing patients' management preferences.
- Loss of decision-making capacity can occur rapidly with the onset of respiratory failure.
- Patients with chronic non-malignant disease are at particular risk of becoming anxious or depressed because of the typically lengthy and unpredictable trajectory.
- Breathlessness and the fear of dying acutely breathless or choking can lead to significant distress, and concerns that are challenging to articulate.
- Misconceptions about advanced non-malignant disease are common, such as lack of recognition of the progressive and life-limiting nature of the disease.

Advance care planning discussions may need to be initiated earlier than in many other advanced diseases. Communication in relation to prognosis in chronic non-malignant disease is particularly challenging.

Key skills

A framework for effective communication, based on the Calgary Cambridge model[1] is outlined in Table 8.2. Discussion of prognosis and advance care planning require particular focus on the following process skills.

Listening
The order in which patients present their concerns does not relate to their clinical importance. Indeed, patients tend to save the most difficult questions until the end. Allowing the patient to complete their narrative without interruption greatly increases understanding of the patient's perspective.

Open questioning

Establishing whether a patient is prepared to discuss prognosis and plan for the future relies on open questioning. Useful phrases include:

- 'How do you feel things are going at the moment?'
- 'What are your greatest fears and concerns for the future?'
- 'What are you hoping we can achieve?'
- 'In your darkest moments…'

Picking up cues

Noticing and responding to both verbal and non-verbal cues can be highly revealing and very effective in improving communication. A patient may, for example, mention concerns about how a spouse is coping, which could be indicative of much greater fears for the future in terms of potential length of life and place of care.

- 'You mentioned feeling upset yesterday. What are the biggest worries on your mind at the moment?'
- 'Yes, it is frustrating not being able to make plans, isn't it? How do you feel things are going at the moment? Would you like to talk about what may be ahead?'
- 'You mentioned about when your mother was dying. Are you worrying about this in relation to you?'

Using a 'dual approach'

A well-established technique in discussions relating to the end of life is to take the dual approach of encouraging and sharing hope, while also making plans and preparing for death:[2,3]

- 'I encourage you to hope for and expect the best, but it is also wise to prepare for the worst.'
- 'I share your hope, and we will do our very best to keep things as good as possible. But it's hard to predict the future, and I imagine you would not want to leave all responsibility for making decisions to your family if you suddenly became very sick. Shall we take a few minutes to think about decisions you might want to make in advance?'

Avoiding unhelpful phrases

A number of phrases are regularly used without appreciation of the devastating impact the words may actually have:

- 'Nothing more can be done…'
- 'Stopping treatment…'
- 'Withdrawing care…'

These phrases should be avoided. It should be made clear that limiting potentially life-sustaining treatment, such as CPR or NIV for example, does not equate with limiting care. 'Not for resuscitation' does not mean 'not for active treatment…' Patients with advanced disease inevitably feel a degree of abandonment. It is vital not to compound this with insensitive communication. Be explicit in your explanations:

- 'We are not going to give up trying to help you. Although we cannot change what this disease is doing, we will do our best to help you live with it, with as good a quality of life as possible.'

Improving communication skills

Most communication skills are acquired in the first few years of practice, when perceived time pressures can discourage patient-centred communication. Although some people have a natural ability to communicate well, there is clear evidence that communication skills are not simply innate. They can be learned and improved.

Communication skills courses provide research evidence on the importance of good communication skills, demonstrate the skills to be learned, provide an opportunity to practise the skills, and give constructive feedback on performance. There is evidence that communication skills training can change a clinician's behaviour and improve communication.

In the UK, a national programme for advanced communication skills has been developed. This offers a 3-day training course for senior health professionals working with patients with cancer. See *www.connected.nhs.uk* for further details.

Mr G was a 65-year-old man with lung cancer. He was admitted with a chest infection and recovered slowly. This was his third chest infection over the last 2 months. On a ward round prior to discharge, the doctor asked him how he felt things were going overall.

Mr G: 'I don't know, and I don't want to know. I just want to get out of here.'

Doctor: 'I can see you are feeling upset. And I can understand that there must be a lot on your mind at the moment. What are you finding the single hardest thing at the moment?'

Mr G: 'My wife has always relied on me for everything, and she won't cope if I'm not there. And don't you go telling her what is going to happen.'

Doctor: 'You are clearly feeling that the future is not looking good... I've noticed your wife looking very tearful in the corridor the last couple of days. I haven't talked to her about your condition, as we had not agreed that I could. But I do get the impression she knows what is happening, and is feeling rather scared. It is quite common for people to feel very alone at this sort of time, because everyone tries to protect each other by not talking about what the future might hold.'

Mr G: 'You mean she might know and isn't talking about it because she doesn't want to upset me...? I didn't think she knew...'

Doctor: 'I suspect if you gently brought up talking about how things are going with her, you'd find you've been thinking about many of the same things. Neither of you would then be alone in your own worries during this uncertain and difficult time...'

Mr G did indeed choose to talk more openly with his wife that evening. The next day he shook the doctor's hand warmly as he left the ward.

'I'm so grateful to you. We're in this one together and stronger for it. And we've decided to take a trip to our caravan this spring while the going is good...'

Table 9.1 Framework for effective communication (adapted from the Calgary Cambridge model)

Task	Skills	Comments and evidence
Initiating the session: • establishing initial rapport • identifying reasons for consultation	• Listen without interruption. • Summarize main problems and screen for others. • Negotiating agenda.	• Doctors interrupt patients after a mean time of only 23 seconds. • Most patients who are allowed to complete their opening statement take less than 60 seconds.[4]
Gathering information: • exploration of problems • understanding the patient's perspective	• Encourage patient's narrative. • Use an 'open to closed' cone of questioning. • Pick up on cues, both verbal and non-verbal. • Clarification of understanding. • Internal summarizing. • Establish time frame and sequence of events. • Encourage expression of ideas, concerns, feelings, expectations.	• Start with open questions. Later on, focus on areas of interest with increasingly closed questions. • Summarize information to show patients they have been heard and to give them the opportunity to correct misunderstandings. • Encouraging patients to be exact about the sequence in which events occurred helps aids recall and helps patients feel understood. • Consider feeding back intuition, such as 'You say that you're managing, but I get the impression you are struggling on some levels with all you are having to cope with.' • 'Blocking behaviour' from clinicians includes early offering of advice and reassurance, focusing on physical aspects, explaining away distress as normal, and 'jollying' patients along.
Explanation and planning: • providing the correct amount and type of information • aiding accurate recall and understanding • achieving a shared understanding • shared decision-making	• Avoid use of jargon. • Increase recall with summarizing, repetition, clarity, and use of diagrams or written summaries. • Ask patients to repeat information in own words. • Establish explicitly whether patients wish to be involved in decision-making. • Give the range of options and discuss pros and cons of each.	• Recall of information is particularly poor immediately after bad news has been received. Try to limit the amount of information given and focus on key messages. • Higher levels of negotiation or participation in the decision-making process lead to increased satisfaction and compliance. • Not all patients wish to be involved in decision-making. This may be decision-specific, and wishes should be established with each important decision. • Avoid giving too many options. Explain and provide a rationale for any recommended options.

(Continued)

Table 8.2 (Continued)

Task	Skills	Comments and evidence
Closing the session: • ensuring appropriate point of closure • forward planning	• Summarize again. • Make contract regarding next steps. • 'Safety netting'—explaining possible unexpected outcomes and when and how to get help. • Final checking—check they agree with plan and give opportunity for final questions.	• 'Safety netting' is particularly important for those with advanced disease. • Open-ended follow-up appointments should be accompanied with clear instructions about how to make an urgent appointment. Be aware that patients may misinterpret a lack of routine follow-up as evidence of abandonment.
Throughout consultation: • building a relationship • providing structure and flow	• Use appropriate non-verbal behaviour. • Non-judgemental, empathetic, supportive attitude. • Involve patient, sharing thinking and explaining rationale. • Progress from one section to another using sign-posting and transitional statements. • Attend to timekeeping.	• There is clear research evidence that building a rapport with patients increases patient satisfaction and compliance. • Sign-posting near the beginning of the consultation that the clinician wishes to consider advance care planning can help patients be prepared for this when the topic arises. • An example of a transitional statement: 'We have been discussing how we are looking after you currently. I wonder whether you would like to go on to talk about how you would like us to look after you in the future?'

References

1. Kurtz SM, Silverman JD, Draper J (1998) *Teaching and Learning Communication Skills in Medicine*. Radcliffe Medical Press (Oxford).
2. Back A, Arnold R, Quill T. 2003. Hope for the best, and prepare for the worst. *Ann Intern Med*, 138:439-43.
3. Hansen-Flaschen J. 2004. Chronic obstructive pulmonary disease: the last year of life. *Respir Care*, 49:90-7.
4. Beckman H, Frankel R. The effect of physical behaviour on the collection of data. *Ann Int Med* 1984, 101: 692-6.

Sharing bad news

'Break bad news well and you will always be remembered; break bad news badly and you will never be forgotten.'

Oxford Handbook of Palliative Care 2005

Breaking bad news to patients and their families can be challenging and stressful. It is the form of communication that clinicians tend to dread most. However, bad news can only be judged 'in the eye of the beholder', and the impact of the news is greatly influenced by the recipient's existing understanding and expectations.

It is unusual for patients with advanced, progressive disease to have no concept at all of the life-limiting nature of their condition, although they may well have chosen not to discuss it, or even tried to deny it. In practice, bad news given with compassion and encouragement of realistic hope tends not to have the devastating impact that one might have envisaged. Bad news discussed is rarely worse than bad news imagined.

Barriers to breaking bad news

Healthcare professionals are uncomfortable breaking bad news for a number of reasons:

- Uncertainty about the patient's expectations.
- Fear of destroying the patient's hope.
- Feeling unprepared to deal with the patient's or family's emotions.
- A sense of failure at being unable to control the progressive disease.
- Embarrassment at having painted too optimistic a picture previously.
- Wanting to avoid a stressful and time-consuming task.

These factors can mean that professionals put off initiating 'bad news' conversations, such as discussion of prognosis. It is vital not to allow these barriers to hinder communication. There is clear evidence that patients want to be told the truth about their illness and prognosis. Without honest communication it is not possible to plan for the future. A patient may therefore die without having had time to prepare for death, leaving family shocked by the unanticipated turn of events.

A framework for sharing bad news

The process of breaking bad news should be a flexible process that is tailored to the individuals concerned. The following framework provides a basis that can be adapted according to each set of circumstances.

Prepare carefully

- Be as well informed as possible about the clinical situation, including previous information given and the patient's response.
- Arrange a comfortable and private environment, with tissues available.
- Make sure there is sufficient time available and take steps to avoid interruptions, such as turning off pagers or mobile phones.
- Particularly if time is relatively limited, ensure a colleague with more time is able to join the conversation, staying with the patient afterwards to provide continuing support.

- Invite family or friends as appropriate, giving the patient the choice. Where there are many family members, ask the patient to choose one or two representatives.

Gather information

Sharing bad news tends to be thought of as information giving rather than receiving, and it is easy to omit this step. This is, however, arguably the most important step of all. Without this, communication cannot be tailored to the individual, and is far more likely to result in distress that could have been so easily avoided.

- Always establish the patient's understanding of the situation first. Try to find out what they already know, and their beliefs and expectations.
- Ask the patient how much they wish to know. A question such as 'Are you the type of person who likes to know what is happening (or wants detailed information)?' can be very revealing. Patients who do not invite further discussion may agree to an offer to speak to family instead.

Share information
- Give a 'warning shot' that potentially difficult information is coming, such as 'I'm afraid the news is less good than we had hoped.'
- Give the basic information simply and clearly. Avoid jargon entirely, and repeat the important points.
- Speak honestly but sensitively, avoiding excessively blunt turns of phrase.
- Give information in small 'chunks', pausing to check understanding periodically.
- Relate the information to the patient's existing understanding and beliefs.

Respond to the patient
- Gauge carefully the patient's need for further information. Most people are unable to absorb further information if the news has been unexpectedly bad. Give time and space if a patient 'shuts down' and stops listening.
- Encourage expression of feelings, if necessary giving explicit encouragement: 'How does this leave you feeling?'
- Respond to any emotional reaction (disbelief, denial, crying, anger) with empathy: 'I know this isn't what you wanted to hear. I wish the news were better.' 'I can see how upsetting this is for you.'
- Try to find out the reason for the patient's emotional response. For example, news of a short prognosis may lead to sadness not at the thought of dying, but at the prospect of being a burden on a spouse.
- Check the patient's understanding of the information that has been given: 'Would you like to run through what you might want to tell your family?'
- Avoid becoming too upset, as this inappropriately burdens the patient with trying to protect the news-giver. However, subtle non-verbal evidence that the professional is feeling saddened can be supportive.

Planning and support
- Try to develop a plan with clear future steps. This can reduce anxiety and uncertainty. It may be necessary to do this in a subsequent consultation, ideally not that long after the initial conversation.
- Foster realistic hope by considering what it is possible to accomplish, such as good control of symptoms, ability to attend an important family event etc.
- Discuss and arrange future support. Patients tend to feel isolated and fearful after having received bad news, and continued support from familiar members of their healthcare team is of great value.
- Document the content of the discussion clearly. A summarizing letter written to the general practitioner should be copied to the patient. Consider giving the patient other written information in addition.

Communicating with carers

'Patient and caregiver information needs show a tendency to diverge as illness progresses, with caregivers needing more and patients wanting less information.'

Parker et al. (2007)[1]

In the UK, over 50% of complaints received by the independent regulator of healthcare relate to care at the end of life. The commonest source of complaint is poor communication, usually with family members.

General principles relating to communication with carers are given below. Specific communication needs of families in the terminal phase are detailed in Chapter 12, and further guidance about family support and bereavement care is given in Chapter 14.

Confidentiality

Always respect patient confidentiality. Communication should not occur with family members unless the patient has given explicit consent for this to happen, either concurrently or in the recent past. The only exception is where the patient does not have the capacity to give consent. In such situations, it is usually in the patient's best interest for communication to occur with family.

Try to gain consent for family members to be included in important discussions with patients from the start. If patients do not wish to discuss their disease or undertake advance care planning, or if they ask for family not to be included in such discussions, their views should be respected.

In practice, however, it is rare for a patient to continue to withhold consent for communication with carers if it is sensitively explained that the family member would find it easier to cope if their questions and concerns could be addressed. Should consent still not be forthcoming, gently explore the reasons for the patient's approach.

Patients may fear that open communication with a fragile family member would lead to distress and breakdown. Address such concerns compassionately, including explanation that imagined fears are often even worse than reality. Patients approaching the end of life tend to be greatly reassured when they understand that the healthcare team is taking on responsibility for supporting their close family.

It is ideal for communication with carers to occur during conversations with the patient, so that all parties are privy to the same information. However, there can also be a place for communication with family alone, with consent, as this may allow the family member to speak more openly than he/she would feel comfortable doing in front of the patient.

Early and explicit communication

Two important features of advanced respiratory disease lead to the need for early and clear communication with family members:

- High frequency of misconceptions about the progressive nature of chronic non-malignant respiratory disease such as COPD.
- Unpredictable trajectory, with typically sudden and unanticipated decline in the terminal phase.

Actively seek out and address misconceptions about the patient's disease. Whereas with advanced malignant disease, hints such as 'things are not going that well' may be understood, in non-malignant disease it may still not occur to family members that the condition will be life-limiting.

Explain that the difficulty in predicting prognosis means that it is worth being prepared for a wide range of future outcomes, from relatively stable disease to rapid deterioration and unexpectedly early death. This both fosters hope, while also preparing for the worst.

Mrs S complained to the local hospital about the care her late husband had received during his final admission. Mr S had had three admissions to hospital during the winter, with infective exacerbations of COPD. Each time he had recovered with IV antibiotics, and she had assumed the same would occur this last time. However, he became very agitated one night, and a doctor phoned her and said that she 'had to come quickly'. Within minutes of her arrival he stopped breathing, and she was horrified that no one attempted to resuscitate him. She screamed at the healthcare team to 'do something' and was told it was 'too late'.

She said in her letter of complaint that no one had ever told her that he might die from his 'bronchitis' and she was sure he would have wanted the doctors to treat him more actively. If they had known how ill he was, they would not have just sold their house and would have planned the last few months very differently, including taking a holiday in their favorite resort on the south coast. Now, several months on, she was still locked in despair, with regular nightmares relating to the events of the last minutes of her husband's life.

Significant event analysis led to the following insights and outcomes:
- No healthcare professional had taken responsibility for discussing prognosis and advance care planning with Mr and Mrs S. The community primary care team had assumed the hospital respiratory team would do this, and vice versa.
- It was decided that the respiratory nurse specialist team would take overall responsibility, and training in advanced communication skills was made mandatory.
- The respiratory nurse specialist team was reconfigured to give more time for outreach domiciliary visits, to create better opportunities for advance care planning discussions to occur at home.
- An audit of the hospital resuscitation policy was undertaken, to ensure that all resuscitation decisions were discussed with patients and their family (other than in exceptional circumstances where such a conversation was believed to be likely to cause harm).

Reference

1. Parker S, Clayon J, Hancock K *et al.* (2007) A systematic review of prognostic/end of life communication with adults in the advanced stages of a life-limiting illness: patient/caregiver preferences for the content, style, and timing of information. *J Pain Sy Manage*; 34 (1): 81–93.

Communicating within healthcare teams

Patients with advanced respiratory disease are cared for by a wide range of health carers from a number of disciplines, across several settings. Accurate sharing of information under such circumstances can be a considerable challenge.

• Weekly multidisciplinary team meetings in inpatient settings are vital. These provide a forum for debate, as well as communication of facts. The outcomes of discussion must be recorded in the patient's notes.
• Discharge and clinic letters should be copied to key professionals across all settings, as well as to the patient.
• Information technology can facilitate accurate and speedy communication across settings. In the UK, technology is being developed for electronic patient summary records to be stored on a national Care Records Service, accessible across all settings.
• Link nursing roles between community and inpatient settings can play an important part in ensuring sharing of information and continuity of care.
• Communication can be enhanced by having a patient 'key worker', providing a single point of contact for the patient and other healthcare professionals. Respiratory nurse specialists working across community and hospital settings can be well placed to fill this role. See 📖 Chapter 10, p. 216 for further details.

Further reading

Advance care planning: a guide for health and social care staff. http://www.endoflifecareforadults. nhs.uk/assets/downloads/pubs_Advance_Care_Planning_guide.pdf.

Baile W, Buckman R, Lenzi R et al. (2000) SPIKES – a six step protocol for delivering bad news: application to the patient with cancer. *The Oncologist*; 5: 302–311.

Barnes K, Jones L, Tookman A, King M (2007) Acceptability of an advance care planning interview schedule: a focus group study. *Palliative Medicine*; 21: 23–28.

Dying Matters Coalition website: http://www.dyingmatters.org/

Steinhauser K, Clipp E, McNeilly M et al. (2000) In search of a good death: observations of patients and providers. *Annals of Internal Medicine*; 132: 825–832.

Further reading

Ethical and legal considerations

Principles of ethical decision-making

Healthcare professionals are frequently confronted by ethical dilemmas when caring for patients with advanced respiratory disease. Many clinical decisions involve an ethical as well as a scientific component. An ability to use ethical reasoning to decide upon an appropriate course of action is as important a skill as that of being able to undertake evidence-based scientific reasoning.

A degree of skepticism about ethical decision-making can occur because such reasoning is based on personal and societal values, rather than on empirical fact. Moral matters never have an absolutely right or wrong answer; they are simply subjective opinion. Thankfully, however, ethical decision-making is invariably easier in practice than in theory. Professionals operate in a national legal framework, which incorporates current societal ethical standards. Furthermore, guidelines from organizations such as the General Medical Council (GMC) in the UK provide explicit guidance as to how professionals are expected to behave.

Bioethical principles

Four key principles have been identified that can clarify the moral issues involved and so contribute to decision-making. The principles of doing good (beneficence) without doing harm (non-maleficence) form arguably the earliest principles of medical ethics, espoused originally by Hippocrates in the 5th century BC.

Beneficence
This principle emphasizes the importance of doing good to others. It raises the question of who is able to judge what is best for a patient.

Non-maleficence
The importance of not harming others needs to be balanced against beneficence. Medical interventions may do both good and harm; the severity and probability of each must be weighed up in order to decide what is in a patient's best interests overall.

Respect for autonomy
Respect for the individual has informed the development of patient-centred medicine, and requires professionals to help patients make their own decisions.

Justice
This principle deals with the importance of any action being fair or just to those in the wider community. Respect for individual autonomy needs to be balanced with fairness at a societal level.

Types of ethical decisions in end of life care

The most challenging and sensitive decisions in this context relate to the following issues:

- Determining the best interests of those without the capacity to make a specific decision themselves.
- Withholding or withdrawing potentially life-prolonging treatments.
- Confidentiality, truth-telling, and collusion.

Framework for ethical decision-making

- Identify the ethical issue(s).
- Gather the following information:
  - medical and social facts
  - relevant values of the patient and family
  - professional guidelines (e.g. GMC)
  - national legal context.
- Find solution(s) consistent with facts, values, guidelines, and law.
- When there is more than one solution, explain the options to the patient.
- Consider recommending a particular option with justification of choice.
- Allow the patient to make a choice, which may include:
  - selection of a preferred option
  - requesting that the professional should make the decision
  - asking for a second opinion.

Legal context

In the UK, a body of statute and case law incorporates current ethical standards and facilitates ethical decision-making at the end of life. Although readers from other countries will not necessarily be bound by equivalent legislation, a summary of existing UK law may be of value in guiding ethical decision-making irrespective of the setting.

Human Rights Act 1998

This Act incorporates into UK law the majority of the rights set out in the European Convention on Human Rights. The rights most relevant to those caring for patients at the end of life are as follows:

- Article 2—the right to life, and a positive duty on public authorities to protect life.
- Article 3—the right to be free of inhuman or degrading treatment.
- Article 8—the right to respect for private and family life.
- Article 9—the right to freedom of thought, conscience, and religion.
- Article 14—the right to be free from discrimination in the enjoyment of other rights in the Act.

The Act has had less impact on medical law than anticipated, as it is broadly consistent with established case law and professional guidance. Of importance, however, is that it allows courts to consider both a decision and the decision-making process. It is particularly important that the process of making ethical decisions is transparent and recorded in detail.

Mental Capacity Act 2005 (England and Wales)

This Act applies to those over the age of 16 and aims to empower and protect vulnerable people who may be unable to make their own decisions. It is underpinned by five key principles:

- A presumption of capacity—every adult has the right to make his or her own decisions and must be assumed to have capacity to do so unless it is proven otherwise.
- The right for individuals to be supported to make their own decisions—people must be given all appropriate help before a conclusion can be taken that they lack capacity.
- Individuals must retain the right to make decisions that could be seen as unwise or eccentric.
- Best interests—anything done for or on behalf of people without capacity must be in their best interests.
- Least restrictive intervention—anything done for or on behalf of people without capacity should be the least restrictive of their basic rights and freedoms.

The Act sets out a clear test to determine mental capacity, and contains a checklist of factors that must be considered in order to determine a patient's best interests (see 📖 pp. 198–201). It also allows patients to create an advance decision to refuse treatment (ADRT), or to appoint a lasting power of attorney (LPA) (see 📖 p. 202).

Case law

Although healthcare professionals have a duty to protect life, a number of legal judgements have shown that the courts do not always consider that protecting life must take precedence over other considerations. A number of important principles established in law are relevant to the care of those near the end of life.

- An act where the doctor's primary intention is to bring about death would be unlawful.
- A competent adult may decide to refuse treatment even when that refusal may lead to harm to themselves or their own death. Doctors that object to the decision are duty bound to find another doctor that will carry out that patient's wishes.
- Life-prolonging treatment may lawfully be withheld or withdrawn from incompetent patients when commencing or continuing treatment is not in their best interests.
- There is no obligation to give treatment that is futile or burdensome.
- If a patient requests a treatment that a doctor has not offered and the doctor concludes that the treatment will not provide overall clinical benefit to the patient, the doctor is not obliged to provide it, although s/he should offer to arrange a second opinion.
- Where artificial nutrition or hydration is necessary to keep a patient alive and a competent patient wishes to receive it, the duty of care will normally require the doctor to provide it.
- Artificial nutrition and hydration may be withheld or withdrawn where the patient does not wish to receive them, or when the patient is dying and the care goals change to palliation of symptoms and relief of suffering, or in patients that lack capacity where such intervention is not considered to be in their best interests.

Assessment of mental capacity

In the UK, the Mental Capacity Act (2005) provides the legal criteria for lack of capacity and the approach to assessment of best interests. Although law will vary between countries, the Act provides a useful framework, irrespective of country of practice.

Assessment of mental capacity

A person lacks capacity to make a decision if he or she 'is unable to make a decision for himself... because of an impairment of, or a disturbance in, the functioning of the mind or brain.'

> A person is unable to make a decision if he or she is unable to do one or more of the following:
> • Understand the information relevant to the decision.
> • Retain the information.
> • Use or weigh that information as part of the process of making the decision.
> • Communicate the decision.

The following points should be considered when assessing the mental capacity of a patient to make a decision.
• Capacity to make a decision is decision-specific. It is possible to have the mental capacity to make one decision, while at the same time lacking the capacity to make another decision.
• The standard of proof of capacity is based on 'the balance of probabilities' rather than 'beyond all reasonable doubt'. The assessment of capacity should determine whether the balance of probabilities favours capacity or lack of capacity.
• A patient should be assumed to have capacity unless proven otherwise. The onus of proof lies with showing that someone lacks rather than has capacity.
• An unwise or eccentric decision is not in itself sufficient grounds to consider that a patient lacks capacity to make the decision. An unwise decision can only alert a doctor to the need to assess mental capacity.
• The fact that a person may only be able to retain information for a short period of time does not in itself imply lack of capacity to make a decision.
• Mental capacity is ultimately a legal not a medical decision, and it is for a court of law to make the final decision. However, in practice, courts take considerable notice of doctors' assessments of patient capacity.

Patients should be given all appropriate help to enhance their capacity to make a decision. The following may be necessary:
• Using simple language, written information, or diagrams.
• Looking for and treating reversible causes of confusion, such as a chest infection.
• Using hearing aids and communication aids.
• If capacity fluctuates, assessing capacity and trying to make the decision at the time a patient is at his/her best.

- Choosing an environment that maximizes capacity, for example with minimal distractions.
- Allowing a person time to make a decision.

Mrs P is a 56-year-old lady with advanced lung cancer, diabetes, and renal failure. She is becoming progressively less well and her husband has been told that her prognosis is measured in weeks only. Her condition deteriorates acutely and she is admitted to hospital, anuric and comatose. It becomes apparent that she now has acute on chronic renal failure and has developed toxicity from the opioids she uses for chest pain. She is not a candidate for dialysis and you expect her to die in the next few days. Her husband becomes distressed and he says she has recently mentioned a wish to die at home. What will you do?

Due to her extremely poor condition you do not think a transfer home would necessarily be in her best interests, as she might die during the journey home. You try to enhance her capacity to make the decision herself. You give her a small dose of intravenous naloxone as her respiratory rate has dropped to six breaths per minute. She wakens fully for an hour, and is able to have a rational and frank discussion about her situation. She clearly reiterates her wish to die at home, and is prepared to take the risk of dying in the ambulance. You therefore arrange for her to be transferred quickly home, under the care of her GP and community specialist palliative care services. She dies at home in a bed with a view over her beloved garden. Her husband writes to you to express his gratitude.

Assessment of best interests

When a patient lacks capacity, there are three main approaches that can be taken to make the decision:
1. Deciding what would be in a patient's best interests.
2. Using a proxy to make the decision.
3. Using an advance decision.

When a patient lacks capacity, the decision is most commonly made by considering what would be in their best interests. Use of a proxy decision-maker or a formal advance decision occurs less often and is described on page 202.

At the core of a decision about a patient's best interests must be a sound clinical judgement, which is based on an assessment of prognosis, the likely benefits and burdens of treatment options, and possibly the opinion of a colleague with relevant expertise.

A number of other factors must also be taken into account when assessing the best interests of a patient:
• the patient's past and present wishes and feelings, including any relevant written statements
• the patient's beliefs and values
• any other factors that would have influenced the patient's own decision-making.

The healthcare professional assessing the patient's best interests should proactively gather and consider the views of family members, partners, and carers. It is important to understand that the purpose of this is to obtain evidence in relation to the patient's wishes, beliefs, and values, rather than to find out their personal opinion on the decision in question.

Even though the patient lacks capacity, he/she should still be involved in the decision-making process as much as is possible. Where more than one option seems reasonable in a patient's best interests, the one that least restricts the patient's future choices and freedoms should be chosen.

Note: General Medical Council guidance, 'Treatment and care towards the end of life: good practice in decision making ' (2010), introduced the phrase 'overall benefit' in place of 'best interests'. These two terms may be used interchangeably.

Mr G is an 83-year-old man with end-stage COPD. He develops a chest infection and becomes rapidly more breathless with a severe cough. He is admitted to hospital in a very confused state and his elderly wife tells you that he would not want treatment. She asks you just 'to keep him comfortable'. What will you do?

His son has now arrived, and you find out more from both family members. Until four days ago Mr G had a reasonably good quality of life and was managing to keep gently active in the garden. He had never talked about wanting to die until the day before admission when, after his third night of little sleep, he said to his wife that 'he wanted it all to be over'.

You decide that it would be in his best interest to commence antibiotics. His recent statement is likely to have been influenced by his acutely unwell state.

He responds reasonably well to antibiotics and is discharged home after a week. His respiratory nurse specialist meets him at home a week later to discuss his wishes regarding treatment and care in the future.

Comment: In hospital, the least restrictive treatment option was chosen, and the use of antibiotics helped improve Mr G's own capacity to make decisions. The subsequent advance care planning discussion was a relief to him and his wife, who now feel calmer and more in control.

Advance and proxy decisions

When a patient anticipates lacking capacity to make a healthcare decision in the future, it is possible to influence the decision made in a number of ways. The patient can tell people what their future wishes and preferences are, or write them down in a statement. Healthcare professionals can use this information to help them ascertain what decision would be in the best interests of the patient should they lack capacity. Chapter 8 describes the process of advance care planning in more detail.

The patient may also influence future decisions by a) making a formal decision to refuse treatment, or b) appointing a proxy trusted to make that decision should the need arise. In the UK, the legal basis for these two options is contained in the Mental Capacity Act (MCA, 2005). Although specific to the UK, the principles described below form a framework that can be used to guide practice in other countries.

Advance decision to refuse treatment

An advance decision to refuse treatment (ADRT) is a decision to refuse specified medical treatment should a patient lack capacity in the future. It is made at a time when the patient has capacity and allows extension of a patient's autonomy to a time when he or she lacks capacity. An advance decision can refuse but not demand treatment.

If the ADRT covers treatment that could be 'life-sustaining':
• It must be in writing, signed, and witnessed.
• It must expressly state that it applies 'even if life is at risk', a statement that must also be signed and witnessed.

In practice, the usefulness of an ADRT is limited by the fact that it can often be invalid. An ADRT is not valid or applicable if:
• It does not relate to the specific treatment/circumstances in question.
• Any circumstances specified in the ADRT are absent.
• The patient has withdrawn the decision orally or in writing at a time when he/she had the capacity to do so.
• The patient has appointed a proxy decision-maker (see below).
• The patient has since behaved in a manner inconsistent with the ADRT.
• There are reasonable grounds for believing that circumstances now exist that the patient did not anticipate at the time of the ADRT, and that would have affected the decision had they been known.

When an ADRT is not valid, it can still be used to guide a decision about what would be in a patient's best interests.

Lasting power of attorney

The MCA allows a patient to create a lasting power of attorney (LPA) that gives authority to a chosen person (an attorney) to make decisions about any specified matters of personal welfare, should the patient lack capacity in the future. An attorney can only give consent to carry out or continue life-sustaining treatment if this has been expressly stated at the time the power was given. An LPA must be registered with the Office of the Public Guardian in order to be valid.

Withholding and withdrawing treatment

Principles

Treatment can be withheld or withdrawn in the following situations:

- It cannot benefit the patient, or the burden of treatment outweighs the likely benefit.
- It has been refused by a patient (with the capacity to make that decision) or is not in accord with a valid advance decision to refuse treatment.
- It is considered not to be in the best interests of a patient who lacks capacity to make a decision regarding treatment.

A broad international consensus states that there is no ethical difference between not starting (withholding) and stopping (withdrawing) treatment. The undoubted emotional difference, it feeling inherently easier to withhold than to withdraw treatment, has led to ongoing debate. In practice, however, creating a distinction between the two would have dangerous consequences, with treatments being continued for too long. A justification for not commencing a treatment must also be sufficient for ceasing it.

The ethical principles and legislation described on pp. 194–197 give clear guidance as to what to do in most situations. Importantly, the first step must always be to assess a patient's capacity to make a decision about treatment. The test for capacity is described on pp. 198–199.

Patient with capacity

- Refuses treatment that the doctor wants to give:
  - Even if refusal may result in death, treatment cannot be given.
- Requests treatment that the doctor does not want to give:
  - The doctor has no obligation to give futile treatment or treatment where s/he believes the burdens will outweigh the benefits. If the situation is not clear-cut, a second opinion should be offered.

Patient without capacity

- A doctor is obliged to act in the patient's best interests, taking into account the medical and social context, and the previous views and wishes of the patient (see pp. 200–201).
- A valid advance decision to refuse treatment or a lasting power of attorney will have a legally binding influence on the decision (see p. 202).

Practical examples

The four treatments that may most commonly be withheld or withdrawn in patients with advanced respiratory disease are:

- antibiotics for a chest infection
- ventilation for respiratory failure
- intravenous hydration and nutrition
- cardiopulmonary resuscitation in the event of cardiopulmonary arrest.

Antibiotics

Antibiotics are usually reasonably effective at treating infection, and are generally not a significant burden (other than the need for hospital admission for intravenous antibiotics). A decision to withdraw or withhold antibiotics may be made in a number of circumstances, including the following:

• The patient's condition is deteriorating despite maximal use of antibiotics, and escalation to ventilation is not considered appropriate.
• Antibiotics have been ineffective during recent similar deteriorations in condition, and there are no features more suggestive of infection this time.
• A patient with capacity to decide about treatment refuses to start or continue antibiotics.
• A patient who lacks the capacity to decide about treatment has made a valid advance decision to refuse treatment.
• A patient's wishes when s/he had capacity were to have no further antibiotics, and the decision not to start or continue antibiotics is considered to be in his/her best interests now that s/he lacks capacity.

Ventilation

For the majority of patients with advanced, progressive respiratory disease and a poor prognosis, escalation of treatment to invasive ventilation will rarely be in their best interests. Morbidity associated with ventilation is considerable, and includes ventilator-acquired pneumonia and pneumothorax. Weaning patients with advanced disease from ventilation may be a lengthy process, if not impossible.

Decisions about withdrawing ventilation should not occur often, if only patients with a reasonable prognosis and acute, reversible decline are ventilated. Difficulties commonly arise, however, when a patient in acute respiratory distress without capacity to make a decision is unknown to the admitting team. Healthcare professionals must make a rapid decision based on an assessment of the patient's best interests. In practice, the option that is 'least restrictive on a patient's rights or freedoms' (see 📖 pp. 196–197) is for the patient to be ventilated, as not ventilating is likely to lead to death. This clearly demonstrates the importance of advance care planning, with an associated statement of wishes and preferences or an advance decision to refuse treatment.

Short-term non-invasive ventilation (NIV) may be of value even in patients with far-advanced disease during an acute, potentially reversible deterioration, such as that caused by a chest infection. Before such a patient commences NIV, a clear decision should be made and documented as to whether escalation from NIV to invasive ventilation would be appropriate. Withholding or withdrawing NIV may be appropriate in situations that are analogous to the points made above in relation to the use of antibiotics. (See 📖 Chapter 12 pp. 262–263 for a practical approach to withdrawal of ventilation.)

Intravenous hydration and nutrition

Parenteral nutrition is very rarely appropriate in patients with advanced, progressive respiratory disease. There is no evidence that it prolongs life and the burdens are considerable. Decisions about the use of intravenous hydration, however, can be difficult for a number of reasons.

• Drinking is a vital and basic human function and patients are entitled to receive enough fluid to maintain hydration.
• The current evidence about the benefits and burdens of intravenous nutrition is not clear-cut.
• Loss of interest in drink (and food) tends to be inevitable and is a natural process during the terminal phase of life.

Although not evidence-based, there is extensive anecdotal support for the following points.

- Dehydration can cause mild nausea and a distressing sense of thirst.
- Good mouth care, keeping the oral mucosa moist, can greatly diminish, if not stop, the sense of thirst.
- Rehydration in the terminal phase (last few days of life) has the potential to worsen a patient's condition, as membranes function less well and fluid may not stay in the body compartment intended. Patients may develop symptoms including breathlessness, cough, increased sputum production, headache, and ankle or sacral oedema.

A decision may be made to withhold or withdraw parenteral hydration in patients with advanced disease approaching the end of life under the following circumstances:

- It is considered that hydration may cause more harm than benefit in a patient whose death is imminent (in the last hours or days of life).
- A patient with capacity whose death is not imminent decides not to start or continue hydration.
- Hydration is not considered to be in the best interests of a patient lacking capacity whose death is not imminent. The 'best interests' decision may be influenced by the patient's previously expressed wish not to have any intervention to prolong life, or by the view of healthcare professionals that any prolongation of life would cause intolerable suffering. Under the latter circumstances, GMC guidance recommends getting a second opinion from a senior clinician.

A 43-year-old man with small cell lung cancer and brain metastases has been admitted to hospital following progressive deterioration over several weeks, with worsening headache and vomiting. His brain CT scan confirms intracranial disease progression. He is now bed-bound and intermittently drowsy. During the drowsy phases, he stops drinking. His wife is extremely angry that he is 'not being given a drip'. What will you do?

You listen carefully to his wife's concerns. She believes that his life is being shortened by dehydration. She is devastated that her relatively young husband is so unwell, and wants 'something to be done'.

You explain sensitively that his prognosis is now short. She asks to know more and you suggest a prognosis of days to very few weeks. You explain that the drowsiness relates to raised intracranial pressure. The fluctuation in drowsiness may be occurring because the dehydration that occurs when drowsy reduces his intracranial pressure so that he wakens. He then drinks more, becomes more hydrated, his intracranial pressure increases and he becomes drowsy again. You make it clear that parenteral hydration would be likely to increase his drowsiness and would not improve his prognosis. His wife understands and accepts your explanation and is grateful for the frank and compassionate communication.

Comment: If hydration is not in a patient's best interests, parenteral hydration should not be commenced simply to satisfy relatives. On occasion, if hydration is unlikely to do harm, it could be commenced briefly at a slow rate, in order to give relatives time to come to terms with a situation.

Cardiopulmonary resuscitation

Cardiopulmonary resuscitation (CPR) in the event of a cardiopulmonary arrest is a medical treatment like any other. A 'do not attempt resuscitation' (DNAR) decision is a decision to withhold treatment.

In the context of advanced respiratory disease, the most common reason for making a DNAR decision is that CPR would be highly unlikely to be successful ('futile'). Data suggest that patients with cancer or organ failure (including respiratory failure) have a less than 1% chance of surviving a cardiorespiratory arrest. A doctor is not obliged to offer or provide a futile treatment, even at a patient's request.

Successful CPR can be associated with significant morbidity. It can cause complications (such as rib fractures) and may lead to a continuation of life of poor quality and short length. In the small number of patients with advanced disease where CPR may be successful (for example following a cardiac arrhythmia), it may still be considered not to be in a patient's best interests because the harms outweigh the potential benefits.

When CPR is considered to be futile or not in the best interests of a patient, a decision must be made whether or not to inform the patient about the DNAR decision. In general a patient should be informed. However, in some situations it may be unnecessary or, indeed, better for the patient not to discuss CPR:

- When discussions with a patient have made it clear that he/she is accepting and expecting a short prognosis, explicit discussion about CPR is not usually necessary.
- For some patients, particularly if they are anxious or easily distressed, information about interventions that will not be helpful would be unnecessarily burdensome and of little value.

When CPR has a chance of being successful, it may still be withheld in the following situations:

- A patient with capacity decides not to accept CPR following discussion of the potential benefits and burdens of CPR.
- A patient lacking capacity has made a valid advance decision to refuse treatment.

Misconceptions about CPR and DNAR decisions abound. Discussions with patients and their carers should make the following clear.

- A DNAR decision does not equate to 'not for active treatment'. The decision *only* relates to CPR in the event of a cardiopulmonary arrest, and not to other treatments such as intravenous antibiotics.
- The chance of successful resuscitation in patients with cancer or organ failure is less than 1% and, even then, the risks of intervention, in terms of complications or poor post-resuscitation quality of life, can be considerable.

Truth-telling and collusion

'…if there is no truth, there is also no hope.'

FA Shaeffer

There are many occasions between the time of diagnosis and the point of death when 'bad news' may need to be given to a patient. Information about the disease, evidence of progression, and prognosis can all be distressing to receive.

Telling the truth is a moral imperative, and there can be little debate that a patient asking a direct question has a right to expect an honest, albeit compassionate, response. An ethical dilemma can arise, however, when a patient is not asking for information. Should the patient be given the information anyway?

Relatives may gain access to information not known to the patient through a number of routes. The patient may have given consent for relatives to receive information, the patient's confidentiality may have been breached, or disclosing information may have previously been considered to be in the best interests of a patient lacking capacity.

Under such circumstances, relatives not infrequently request that the patient is not given the information, as 'it would make him upset', or 'she would give up hope' or 'die more quickly'. Healthcare professionals that acquiesce with such a request are colluding with the relatives.

The following points can help guide ethical behaviour under these circumstances:

- If a patient with the capacity to decide whether s/he wants information asks to know more, s/he should be told the truth. The information should be given in a sensitive manner as described in Chapter 8.
- A patient has a right to confidentiality. Information should never be given to relatives without the patient's consent unless the patient lacks capacity and it is considered to be in his/her best interests for relatives to be told more.
- Relatives have no right to insist that information about a patient is withheld from the patient. However, understanding a patient's likely reaction to bad news from a relative's perspective can help a clinician decide whether it would be in the best interest of the patient to a) keep quiet and wait for the patient to ask proactively for information, or b) tell the patient that there is some new information and ask him/her whether or not s/he would like to receive it.

In practice, receipt of compassionately given 'bad news' is almost inevitably helpful for a patient. Patients are often far more aware of their predicament than they appear (the impression of being unaware of a poor prognosis may, in fact, occur because the patient is trying to protect relatives). The imagined scenario may be worse than the actual truth. Learning the truth may help the patient develop realistic hope and reasonable plans (for example, hoping and planning to be visited by a close relative who lives abroad), rather than false hope that leads to distress and a sense of failure (such as planning international travel).

Mr M is a 65-year-old widower with end-stage COPD. He is admitted for the sixth time this year with a chest infection. During a previous admission, when he was briefly ventilated, his daughter was told that his prognosis is likely to be short. She begs you not to talk about this with him, as he 'would just give up'. What should you do?

You explain that you will not volunteer unsolicited information, but that if he asks questions, you have a duty to give an honest response. On the day of discharge he mentions to you that he hopes never to see the hospital again. You ask him if he'd like to talk more. He starts to cry and expresses his loneliness: 'I know I'm ill but I can never tell my daughter because she'll not cope'. You compassionately suggest that they may both be 'trying to look after each other' by not talking about the future.

Although his daughter is initially distraught to enter and find her father in tears, their subsequent honest and open conversation allows them to cry together and accept their shared sadness at his deteriorating condition. Mr M reports to his district nurse the following week that he now feels that he can 'live this last part of my life—my daughter and I have just spent the afternoon planning a tea party for family friends.'

Further reading

British Medical Association (2007) *Withholding and Withdrawing Life-prolonging Medical Treatment: Guidance for decision-making.* Blackwell Publishing, Oxford.

British Medical Association, Resuscitation Council (UK), Royal College of Nursing (2007) *Decisions relating to cardiopulmonary resuscitation: A joint statement from the British Medical Association, the Resuscitation Council (UK) and the Royal College of Nursing.* http://www.resus.org.uk/pages/dnar.pdf

General Medical Council (2008) *Consent: Patients and doctors making decisions together.* http://www.gmc-uk.org/static/documents/content/Consent_2008.pdf

General Medical Council (2010) *Treatment and care towards the end of life: good practice in decision making.* http://www.gmc-uk.org/static/documents/content/End_of_life.pdf

Hope T, Savulescu J, Hendrick J (2008) *Medical Ethics and Law.* Churchill Livingstone, Edinburgh

Mental Capacity Act (2005) http://www.opsi.gov.uk/acts/acts2005/pdf/ukpga_20050009_en.pdf

Multidisciplinary working

Introduction

In order to achieve holistic care and meet the complex needs of patients with advanced progressive respiratory disease, teamwork is essential and a multidisciplinary team (MDT) approach is fundamental to ensure the delivery of best quality care. A coordinated approach is of paramount importance, requiring effective liaison between the patient, the patient's family and carers, and health and social work professionals from within the NHS, independent, or voluntary sectors.

There are a number of shortcomings in the current service provision for people with advanced chronic respiratory disease. These include:

- Significant geographical inequalities both within and between countries.
- Disease-specific variations in practice, for example services for patients with lung cancer tend to be better developed than those for patients with COPD, pulmonary fibrosis etc.
- A focus on management of acute exacerbations of disease and prolongation of life, rather than on quality of life.
- A reactive rather than proactive approach to care:
  - Patients may be neglected when not acutely unwell, remaining 'socially invisible' until they enter an acute phase.
  - Emphasis on crisis intervention rather than prevention, with little advanced care planning.
- A fragmented service with inadequate communication between members of the wider MDT, for example between primary and secondary care and between respiratory and palliative medicine services.

In the UK, the National Council for Palliative Care has acknowledged these inequalities. In response, a Chronic Respiratory Disease Policy Group was founded to highlight deficiencies and aid successful implementation of the Department of Health's End of Life Care Strategy recommendations.[1]

Reference

1. The National Council for Palliative Care (2009) *A Fresh Approach: Palliative and end of life care for people with Chronic Respiratory Disease*. www.ncpc.org.uk/policy_unit/circ_resp_pg.html

Principles of service development

Respiratory and primary care services need to integrate palliative care measures for appropriate patients into their routine practice, with close collaboration and support from a local specialist palliative care team.

Mixed management model of care

The traditional model of care of patients with advanced, particularly non-malignant respiratory disease involves a dichotomy, with abrupt transition from active, 'life-prolonging' care to palliative care. This does not work in many advanced respiratory diseases for several reasons:

- The timing of death is unpredictable and it will inevitably be hard to judge when any transition should be made.
- Patients with far advanced disease should not necessarily be denied active intervention, for example ventilatory support during an acute exacerbation.
- Patients may live with a heavy burden of uncontrolled symptoms and psychosocial needs for many years and it would be unethical to deny them good palliation because they are not yet in the end of life phase.

The mixed management model of care is highly appropriate for patients with advanced respiratory disease. Active disease-modifying treatment is combined with good palliative care throughout the disease trajectory. From the time of diagnosis, active management of the underlying disease occurs alongside generalist palliative care measures that improve quality of life.

Principles of service delivery

- High-quality, seamless care should be provided from diagnosis through to bereavement support after death. A whole systems approach is required, matching services to the patient pathway.
- Patient-centred rather than disease-orientated care is vital. A patient-centred approach focuses on maintaining quality of life. Disease-orientated care leads to perceptions of failure as the underlying disease inevitably progresses.
- Care must be provided on the basis of needs rather than on extent of disease. Patients have diverse and complex needs, and care is best provided using the collaborative efforts of a multidisciplinary team.
- Patients live in the community and their care must be based there. Support and prevention during a relatively stable phase can reduce the risk of crises and reactive acute hospital admission.
- Continuity of care is integral to success. Care must be integrated, with coordination between all settings, particularly community and acute hospital teams.
- Close partnership between the patient, families and carers, and health and social care professionals underpins successful service development. Active involvement of patients and carers in decision-making must be supported with the provision of adequate information.
- The effectiveness of services must be monitored. Internal audit, feedback, and appraisal systems can help guide local practice. Formal research evaluation is ideal, comparing patient outcomes before and after creation of a new service model.

The multidisciplinary team

Sustainable service delivery requires a collaborative approach between all members of the multidisciplinary team. A typical team may include:

- A lead physician, usually a respiratory medicine consultant, who takes responsibility for the service.
- Clinical nurse specialists (respiratory, COPD, lung cancer).
- Pulmonary rehabilitation team.
- Volunteers.
- Outpatient services.
- Allied health professionals (see pp. 224–225).
- Hospital and community social workers.
- Specialist palliative care team, including community nurse specialists.
- Team coordinator.
- Secretary (coordinates team, ensures notes are available and decisions accurately documented).

Practicalities of service development

There is consistent evidence that patients with advanced progressive disease want community-based, patient-centred care, with collaboration and integration across all settings. The UK *End of Life Care Strategy*[1] has attempted to achieve this with the development of an end of life care pathway. The components of this pathway are described below, as they show, in practice, how services can be created that meet patient needs.

Care pathway approach

The UK *End of Life Care Strategy* describes a six-step patient pathway (see Figure 10.1).

Discussions as the end of life approaches, including care planning

The 'surprise question' (see 📖 p. 172) is of most value when used by experienced healthcare professionals who can intuitively integrate the myriad of patient factors that impact on prognosis.

- Local service development should identify the staff with sufficient experience to make such a judgement.
- The optimal context, timing, and setting of discussions are described in Chapter 8 (see 📖 pp. 174–176).
- Training in advanced communication skills may be necessary in order that staff feel competent to undertake such conversations.

Delivery of services in different settings and coordination of care

Patients may concurrently access a complex combination of services including, for example, primary care, district nursing, social care services, ambulance/transport services, respite care, out of hours services, occupational therapy, physiotherapy, pharmacy, dietetics, and so on. It is essential that the services are effectively coordinated within teams, between teams, and across organization boundaries. A number of practical measures can help achieve this.

Developing a 'key worker' system

- The MDT appoints a named key worker for each patient in a locality, who provides a single point of contact for the patient. The choice will depend on local service configuration but should ideally be a professional at least partly based in the community. In the UK, staff particularly eligible for the key worker role are the patient's GP, district nurse, or respiratory nurse specialist.
- The key worker is responsible for ensuring patients receive all the information they need, advance care planning, coordinating care between services and settings, and providing a first point of contact.
- Systems must be in place so that the identity and contact details of the key worker can be easily accessed. In the UK, a primary care practice register is often used (see 📖 pp. 230–231).

Use of information technology (IT)

- IT allows rapid, cheap, and accessible sharing of up to date information and can greatly enhance coordination of care.

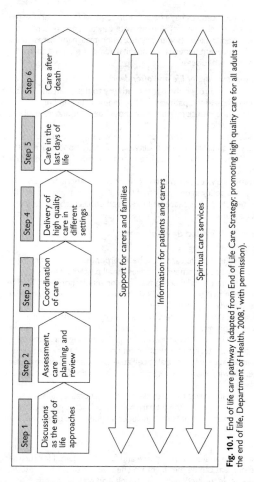

Fig. 10.1 End of life care pathway (adapted from End of Life Care Strategy: promoting high quality care for all adults at the end of life, Department of Health, 2008,[1] with permission).

- A locality-wide register for all those potentially in the last year of life can be set up on a secure IT system. Advance care planning statements may, for example, prevent unnecessary hospital transfer out of hours.

Creating 'link nurse' roles and coordination centres
- A hospital-based community discharge nurse can create vital links between acute hospital and community teams. Such roles increase speed of discharge from hospital and facilitate accurate and speedy sharing of information between sectors.

- Coordination centres have been set up to provide rapid access to care in the community for patients with cancer. This concept can be extended to patients with advanced non-malignant disease and, again, can prevent unnecessary hospital admission during an acute exacerbation of disease.

Care in the last days of life and after death

- Effective care through the patient pathway to this point should facilitate the final steps of the pathway. The patient's wishes and preferences for care, including resuscitation status, should be clear and accessible to all service providers.
- An integrated care pathway for care in the terminal phase of life (last few days) can facilitate high quality care. The Liverpool Care of the Dying Pathway in the UK has been used extensively and is described on ☐ pp. 234–235.
- Innovative services can improve patient/carer experiences. For example, a policy in one region of the UK to train nurses to verify expected deaths has successfully reduced unacceptable delays waiting for a doctor.

Support for service development

Education and training

- Training in end of life care must be incorporated into continuing professional development initiatives for all professionals.
- A priority area is training in advanced communication skills. Staff tend to perceive that they lack the skills to undertake conversations about dying and advance care planning.
- Specialist palliative care services have a key role in developing education programmes and disseminating their expertise. Training is required in all sectors and with all staff, including unregistered staff groups. Integrated education set up by respiratory specialists in collaboration with specialist palliative care teams is of particular value, allowing sharing of expertise and facilitating future collaborative working.
- e-Learning initiatives can provide valuable generalist palliative care education. In the UK, the e-Learning for Healthcare programme run by the Department of Health includes an end of life care e-learning project.[2]

Resources

- Most of the additional workforce and funding required for such service development can be met by more effective use of existing resources. For example, reduction in acute hospital admission can offset the additional costs of providing improved care in the community.
- There is growing international recognition of the importance of providing high quality end of life care, and a number of governments, including that in the UK, are investing in end of life care services. Investment is particularly directed towards non-malignant disease because of the relative paucity of services for such patients in comparison to those with cancer.

- Charitable funding has traditionally supported services for patients with cancer. Charities such as the British Lung Foundation in the UK provide support groups for patients and their carers, but do not develop or support services.

Evaluation and research

- Data collection is vital in order to undertake population needs assessments, to assess the quality and cost-effectiveness of existing and novel services, and for benchmarking between services.
- Quality standards should be developed and evaluated for all services. Measures of patient outcomes and experiences are particularly important, including patient feedback and the results of surveys of patient and carer experiences. Post-bereavement proxy carer surveys are increasingly used to evaluate the care of patients with advanced disease.
- Baseline data should be collected before implementing new services so that the service can be evaluated by comparing pre- and post-service outcomes.

Recommendations of the NCPC[3]:
- Partnership and collaboration is fundamental to meeting the palliative and end of life care needs of people with CRD and their carers.
- Systematic processes must be developed to ensure needs are met:
  - data collection about local population needs and services
  - key stakeholders deciding on a formal process to meet identified needs, including development of a local care pathway
  - user and carer involvement and feedback
  - locality-wide register and other ways of communicating across settings and sectors
  - monitoring and regular evaluation.
- Workforce development should be considered, focusing on key groups of staff such as GPs, respiratory specialist nurses, and respiratory consultants.

Examples of innovative practice

Breathlessness Intervention Service, Cambridge UK

This innovative service is coordinated by a palliative care consultant and a clinical specialist physiotherapist. Patients with intractable breathlessness from any cause are referred from primary and hospital practice. A unique rehabilitative approach is adopted either in a clinic setting or within patients' own homes. Interventions are both non-pharmacological (psychosocial or physical) and pharmacological, and end of life issues and family concerns are also addressed. The clinical effectiveness and cost-effectiveness of this service are currently under evaluation, in a trial randomizing breathless patients between this service and best supportive care.

INSPIRE, Lincolnshire

This specialist respiratory service has developed over the last 10 years. It includes the following:

- Acute respiratory assessment service, seeing patients with acute exacerbations in their own homes.
- Early assisted discharge, aiming to discharge earlier from hospital, giving follow-up care at home and working closely with family.
- After routine discharge, follow-up allows optimization of treatment and referral to other services such as pulmonary rehabilitation.
- Pulmonary rehabilitation, including education in self-management and a session discussing end of life with a consultant psychologist.
- Specialist respiratory physiotherapy in patients' own homes to facilitate breathlessness management and chest clearance.
- Case management for housebound and complex patients.

Respiratory Palliative Care Special Interest Group: the Hospice of St Frances

This group comprises specialist respiratory nurses, community matrons, and respiratory physiotherapists, and is led by a consultant in palliative medicine and an educator who is an expert in communication skills. The meetings empower the respiratory specialist team and community matrons to provide high standards of palliative care and facilitate referrals to specialist palliative care where appropriate. Case-based discussion leads to learning and change in practice, and incorporates evidenced-based practice into everyday clinical care.

Partnership working community matrons, NHS Blackburn

Community matrons case-manage individuals with particularly complex needs, to reduce inappropriate admission to hospital. The team has developed close links with both specialist respiratory and palliative care services, and has jointly developed a care pathway to standardize care provided to those with COPD. The community matron acts as the named nurse for their patients and facilitates joint decision-making and advance care planning.

References

1. Department of Health (2008) *End of Life Care Strategy*. http://www.dh.gov.uk/en/Publications andstatistics/Publications/PublicationsPolicyAndGuidance/DH_086277
2. e-Learning for Healthcare, Association for Palliative Medicine of Great Britain and Ireland (2010) *End of Life Care for All (ELCA): An e-learning project*. http://www.e-lfh.org.uk/projects/e-elca/index. html
3. The National Council for Palliative Care (2009) *A Fresh Approach: Palliative and end of life care for people with Chronic Respiratory Disease*. www.ncpc.org.uk/policy_unit/circ_resp_pg.html

Respiratory and palliative care joint working

Respiratory teams are best placed to provide end of life care for their patients. Although there are pragmatic reasons for this, limited resources meaning that only those with the most complex needs can access specialist palliative services, it is also best practice from the perspective of patients. Patients appreciate continued care from a familiar team that can both optimally manage their disease and provide for their general palliative care needs.

Referral to specialist palliative care services

There are no absolute criteria that determine whether or not to involve specialist palliative care services. As a guide, patients may require the expertise of a specialist palliative care team in the following situations:
- Complex physical needs:
  - Difficulties in gaining or retaining symptom control.
  - Multiple concurrent symptoms.
  - Medical co-morbidity hindering symptom control measures (e.g. renal failure causing opioid accumulation).
- Complex psychosocial or spiritual needs:
  - Significant difficulties adjusting to diagnosis, prognosis, disabilities.
  - Communication problems with professionals or with family.
  - Concerns about children or other vulnerable individuals.
  - Complex practical problems resulting from the illness.
  - Complicated bereavement needs of family.
  - Significant challenge of belief system, faith, or cultural values.

The decision about whether or not to refer to specialist palliative care services will also be influenced by local expertise and resources within the wider respiratory MDT, and also relative capacity in local services.

Specialist palliative care services can provide input at a wide range of levels:
- Telephone advice only on one or more occasions.
- Assessment during acute hospital admission, providing advice to host healthcare team.
- Domiciliary visit by community specialist palliative care team.
- Day hospice care.
- Admission to specialist palliative care unit for control of complex symptoms, psychosocial support, respite care, or terminal care.

Facilitating joint working

Respiratory teams and specialist palliative care teams each have much to contribute to the end of life care of those with advanced respiratory disease. Joint working allows teams with complementary expertise to exchange and share experience, ideas, beliefs, and values, in order to achieve optimal patient care. The emphasis is on 'joined-up' working to achieve a common goal. This type of working can occur in both clinical and academic settings.

Collaborative clinical work

- Joint respiratory/palliative care clinics can work well. The teams learn from each other, and patients can be seen by the professional best placed to meet their needs on that particular day. Patients perceive continuity of care and management from an extended MDT, rather than a dichotomy in care and perception of 'medical failure' that can accompany formal transfer from a respiratory to a palliative care team.
- Significant event debriefing may gain from the expertise of both teams if it relates to, for example, a symptom crisis or other event in the end of life phase.
- Access to 24-hour telephone advice from a specialist palliative care team member (preferably with particular expertise in non-malignant advanced respiratory disease) can empower respiratory teams to provide care throughout the end of life phase.
- An 'end of life care respiratory group' can meet regularly and develop, for example, patient pathways, symptom control guidelines, an advance care planning policy, patient information sheets etc.

Collaborative academic work

- Setting up a joint education programme is an ideal way of sharing expertise, learning from each other, and tackling misconceptions. This could range, for example, from regular lunchtime joint education meetings to an 'end of life care in advanced respiratory disease' conference.
- Research collaboration is of great value. It allows ideas and hypotheses to be shared and developed, builds trust, and can, for example, lead to formal evaluation of end of life care services (see 📖 p. 219).

JF was a 78-year-old man with end-stage COPD. He had been under the care of the respiratory team for 7 years. Over the preceding 3 months, he had had eight hospital admissions with increasing breathlessness and anxiety. His community respiratory nurse specialist visited him and his wife at home and tried to start a conversation about his future wishes and preferences for care. He was, however, defensive and anxious, and became visibly more breathless during the meeting.

The nurse specialist contacted Dr M, a medical member of the local specialist palliative care team, and asked for advice. They undertook a joint domiciliary visit and began to explore the source of his anxiety. They taught him breathing control and relaxation techniques. When the nurse specialist visited a week later, he spontaneously began to talk about his fear of dying acutely breathless with his wife unable to cope.

He agreed to attend a breathlessness clinic run by the respiratory team and specialist occupational therapist. Dr M's telephone advice was sought about appropriate pharmacological interventions for JF's breathlessness and anxiety. JF died 1 month later at home, as he had requested, calm and with his wife beside him, shortly after a joint visit from his district nurse and respiratory nurse specialist.

Contributions from allied health professionals

- Allied health professionals (AHP) are graduate clinicians who play a key role in the provision of end of life care.
- They perform diagnostic and therapeutic tasks across a range of healthcare settings.
- The allied health professionals most involved in the provision of end of life care of patients with respiratory disease include physiotherapists, occupational therapists, and clinical psychologists. Table 10.1 outlines examples of practical input they may provide.
- Other AHP include:
  - art therapists
  - chiropodists/podiatrists
  - diagnostic radiographers
  - dieticians
  - drama therapists
  - orthoptists
  - paramedics
  - prosthetists/orthotists
  - speech and language therapists
  - therapeutic radiographers.
- There is early evidence for a potential role of music therapists in the palliation of breathlessness. Singing requires breathing rate control, prolonged expiration, and diaphragmatic breathing. It is relaxing and sociable. Although its impact on breathlessness remains to be rigorously evaluated, it is a therapy that appears unlikely to cause harm, and should at least be fun!

Table 10.1 Roles of key Allied Health Professionals (AHP)

Physiotherapist	a) Maximise mobility and function. This allows patients to optimise levels of daily functioning and minimise dependency regardless of their life expectancy. Prevention of muscle atrophy and joint contractures will also limit functional decline.
	Practical measures include:
	• Use of appropriate mobility aids
	• Pacing of daily activities: concentrating on important or pleasurable tasks, adapting activities e.g. decreasing housework, accepting external help, and re-arranging time schedules
	• Goal setting for routine daily functional and social activities
	b) Teach non-pharmacologic techniques for the relief of dyspnoea (chapter 5). These include appropriate positioning, pursed lip breathing, relaxation therapy, breathing control advice and retraining, energy conservation and pacing strategies, and distraction devices.
	c) Provide advice and support for patients and their families on ways of managing breathlessness.
	d) Provide an integrated approach in the home (community physiotherapy teams).
Occupational therapist (OT)	a) Assist patients in attaining the occupational roles they perceive to be important, given their limitations of time and physical ability. The ability to perform normal daily living activities is often a primary objective for patients.
	b) Facilitate adaptation of the living environment to anticipate and reduce barriers to functional independence:
	• Limiting unnecessary exertion e.g. moving the bed downstairs
	• Use of selected aids and equipment e.g. commode, hand-rail, tray-mobile walking aids, perching stool.
Clinical psychologist	a) Provide help and support for patients, and their carers, who may find it difficult to cope with the emotional adjustment needed as they strive to adapt to the changes associated with illness - and the need to continue with everyday living.
	b) Provide 'safe' ways to express difficult emotions and support problem-solving skills.
Chaplain	Spirituality and religion are important to patients and families. Leaders of any faith can provide a source of spiritual comfort and a supportive presence for patients and their families. They play a role as listeners, and may have an insight into the religious and cultural factors that can shape how a patient and family face illness and suffering.

Further reading

The National Council for Palliative Care (2009) *A Fresh Approach: Palliative and end of life care for people with Chronic Respiratory Disease.* www.ncpc.org.uk/policy_unit/circ_resp_pg.html

e-Learning for Healthcare, Association for Palliative Medicine of Great Britain and Ireland (2010) *End of Life Care for All (ELCA): An e-learning project.* http://www.e-lfh.org.uk/projects/e-elca/index.html

Department of Health (2008) *End of Life Care Strategy.* http://www.dh.gov.uk/en/Publications andstatistics/Publications/PublicationsPolicyAndGuidance/DH_086277

Department of Health (2008) *Framing the Contribution of Allied Health Professionals.* http://www.dh.gov.uk/en/Publicationsandstatistics/Publications/PublicationsPolicyAndGuidance/DH_089513

Chapter 11

Practical management at the end of life

Introduction

High quality end of life care has a number of important features. The care needs to be:

- patient-centred and responsive to individual needs
- multidisciplinary
- based in the community
- proactive rather than reactive
- integrated across all settings.

Provision of such care is, by definition, a complex process. A potentially large number of professionals in different healthcare settings, from a range of disciplines, and with varied expertise, must coordinate themselves to provide care that is uniquely different for each patient, tailored to individual circumstances and needs.

In recent years, a number of frameworks, tools, and checklists have been developed in the UK in order to facilitate provision of this type of healthcare. These include the Gold Standards Framework (GSF), the preferred priorities for care document (PPC), and the Liverpool Care Pathway for the Dying Patient (LCP), each described in the following pages. These measures are becoming increasingly widely used and are supported by evidence for improved patient outcomes.

Although developed and licensed for use in the UK, international interest is growing and a number of these tools have been adapted for use (under contract) internationally.

Frameworks and other tools can improve the quality of care by supporting, but not by replacing, clinical judgement. Tools are only as effective as the people using them.

Gold Standards Framework

The Gold Standards Framework (GSF) is a common-sense approach to formalizing best practice in caring for patients in the last year of life, and is mainly used within the primary care and care home settings.

The GSF was originally developed in primary care in the UK. Since its first use in 2001 it has been cascaded nationally, with over 90% of general practices adopting at least one level of the GSF. It has been endorsed as best practice across the country and is now central to quality improvement in end of life care.

The core elements of the framework are outlined below. Further details are available at http://goldstandardsframework.nhs.uk.

Three Simple Steps

- **Identify** patients in the last year of life.
- **Assess** current and future clinical and personal needs.
- **Plan** care by developing an action plan.

Seven Key Tasks

- **Communication**: Supportive Care Register (SCR), team planning meetings, advance care plans.
- **Coordination**: identified GSF coordinator, key worker.
- **Control of symptoms**: needs assessment, symptom control.
- **Continuity out of hours**: handover form, out of hours protocol, anticipatory prescribing (see 📖 Chapter 12 p. 260).
- **Continued learning**: reflective practice, significant event analyses, After Death Analysis (ADA) audit tool.
- **Carer support**: practical, emotional, bereavement.
- **Care in the dying phase**: integrated care pathway (LCP, see 📖 pp. 234–235).

Local facilitators work closely with healthcare professionals to set up the elements of the GSF, often starting with a Supportive Care Register and planning meetings. A range of fact-sheets and toolkits are available, as well as accredited training courses and training packs.

Although developed initially in primary care, the GSF includes work streams in care homes (nursing or residential homes) and is being adapted for use in the acute hospital setting.

Evidence

Research and audits have shown three areas of improvement with use of the GSF:

- **Attitude, awareness, and approach**: greater awareness of patient needs, increased confidence and job satisfaction, more focused and proactive approach.
- **Patterns of working, structure, and process**: better organization and consistency, enhanced communication, improved recording and coordination of care, greater collaboration with specialists.

- **Patient and carer outcomes**: reduced hospitalization (crisis admissions reduced by one-third), more home deaths (hospital deaths reduced by half), more advance care planning discussions.

Preferred priorities for care

Advance care planning (ACP) facilitates patients to express their preferences for future care and is an integral component of good quality end of life care. Such planning is of particular importance in patients with advanced respiratory disease; prognosis is uncertain and rapid deterioration during an acute exacerbation can hinder communication at the exact time decisions need to be made (see 📖 Chapter 8, pp. 170–171).

There is clear evidence that ACP discussions are not undertaken as frequently as patients would like. Even when such discussions do take place, decisions recorded in patient notes tend to be either ignored, other professionals being unaware of where to look, or are unavailable to those working in other healthcare settings.

Developing a standardized document to record patients' wishes and preferences for their future care has a number of advantages:
- It may encourage ACP to be undertaken, as the document needs to be completed.
- It can incorporate an information section for patients, ensuring careful explanation of the purpose of the document.
- Standard arrangements can be made for the information to be accessible to professionals across all settings. Electronic sharing of information using a central database is particularly efficient.

Services can develop their own preferred priorities for care (PPC) documentation. In the UK, a standard document has been created by a national PPC review team (available at http://www.endoflifecareforadults. nhs.uk/assets/downloads/ppc.pdf). It contains the following three main questions:
- In relation to your health, what has been happening to you?
- What are your preferences and priorities for your future care?
- Where would you like to be cared for in the future (see Table 12.1 p. 244)?

Although the document is not legally binding, in the event that a patient lacks the capacity to make a decision about his/her care, the information contained in the form would strongly influence future 'best interests' management decisions (see 📖 Chapter 9, pp. 200–201).

Reactive care

Mrs G was an 82-year-old lady with advanced COPD. Whenever she felt less well she called her GP and on several occasions had to be admitted to hospital in the evening by the out-of-hours service. She lived alone and tried to avoid calling her son who was very busy. She wanted to talk about the future but there was never time during consultations.

She became acutely breathless one evening and called an emergency ambulance. After lying on a trolley for 6 hours in the Accident and Emergency department, she was transferred to the ward. Her condition deteriorated rapidly during the night and she then suffered a cardio-respiratory arrest. The on-call medical team tried to resuscitate her without success. Her son was not present, as he had not been aware of how ill she was.

Proactive care

Mr W was a 74-year-old man with rapidly progressing motor neurone disease (MND). His GP was aware of his short prognosis. The GP arranged for Mr W to be entered onto the practice Supportive Care Register and made contact with his MND clinical nurse specialist. She visited Mr W at home, and offered him the opportunity to discuss his concerns about the future. He was relieved to be able to talk openly about his fears, and on her second visit felt able to express his wishes for care when he became less well.

He was visited regularly by his district nurses and when he developed a chest infection they were able to support him, avoiding admission to hospital. He died peacefully at home, with his family around him, as he had wished.

Integrated care pathway

The Liverpool Care Pathway for the Dying Patient (LCP) is a widely used integrated care pathway that was initially developed to extend the excellence of hospice care into the acute hospital setting.

An integrated care pathway is a multidisciplinary care plan that details all the important steps in the care of patients with a specific clinical problem. It is a way of ensuring that agreed guidelines of care are translated into clinical practice.

The LCP is an integrated care pathway that aims to improve the care of patients in the last days or hours of life. It is recognized within the UK as an important component of end of life care quality improvement, as it provides a mechanism for identifying and addressing the needs of dying patients.

The LCP has been adapted for use within a number of specific diagnostic groups, including neurological conditions, heart failure, renal failure, and patients within an intensive care unit. Although not as yet specifically adapted for patients with advanced respiratory disease, the generic version of the LCP remains suitable for use in this patient group.

Core information about the LCP is given below. Further details and supporting information are available at http://www.mcpcil.org.uk.

Using the LCP

The LCP generic version 12 (December 2009) is a 20-page document that replaces the patient's usual healthcare record. It is used when a patient is believed to be in the last days or hours of life.

Recognizing dying

Diagnosis of dying is complex and, on occasion, a patient thought to be dying may live longer than expected.

- The decision to commence the LCP should be taken by the most senior clinician available, with regular multidisciplinary team review at least every 3 days.
- Potentially reversible causes of deterioration in the patient's condition must be considered.
- Factors that can help the diagnosis of dying are described on page 238.

Initial assessment

Goals during the initial assessment include the following:

- The patient and carer/relatives should be aware that the patient is dying.
- The patient should be given the opportunity to discuss what is important to them at this time.
- 'As needed' drugs must be prescribed for a range of symptoms—so-called 'anticipatory prescribing' (see ☐ Chapter 12, p. 260).
- Need for current interventions should be reviewed by the MDT.

Ongoing assessment
- This includes assessment for uncontrolled symptoms, checking psychological well-being, and evaluating the needs of relatives.
- The patient's mouth should be examined to check it is moist and clean, and skin integrity should be assessed.
- If any goals are not achieved in the initial or ongoing assessment, this is recorded as a 'variance' and the reason is recorded and analysed.

Care after death
This section of the LCP includes verification of death and providing information for the relative or carer. It triggers notification of the primary healthcare team and other appropriate services.

Evidence

Evidence from research and audits suggests that the LCP:
- reduces symptom burden
- improves multidisciplinary working
- increases anticipatory prescribing for symptoms that may develop
- improves nurses' confidence in caring for the dying.

There have been anecdotal reports in the UK that use of the LCP, when a patient is incorrectly diagnosed as dying, may actually precipitate death, for example by allowing withdrawal of artificial hydration or inappropriate sedation. There has, however, been no evidence to support these concerns, and the LCP documentation makes it clear that, as with all guidelines and pathways, the LCP aims to support but not replace clinical judgement. If a patient is no longer thought to be in the terminal phase, the LCP can be withdrawn.

Practical issues in the home

Patients with advanced respiratory disease have complex needs that can make living at home challenging. Difficulties include inability to undertake activities of daily living, such as washing and dressing, and the need for significant medical intervention such as oxygen, non-invasive ventilation, and parenteral drug infusions.

Such issues are rarely insurmountable and, with the help of a multidisciplinary team, can usually be overcome. With good home support it is usually possible for patients to be cared for at home, even, if they wish, during the terminal phase.

Difficulties with daily activities

Early and continued occupational therapy assessment is of great importance. A wide range of practical modifications can make it easier for breathless and/or debilitated patients to function at home. For example, wheelchair ramps at any change of level, such as the front door, are often necessary. Replacing a bath with a shower and shower seat, and fixing a stair handrail or stair-lift can also be useful. Alternatively, a hospital-type bed can be installed in a room downstairs. Moving the bed closer to a window and putting a TV set in the room may well be appreciated.

Home oxygen

Ambulatory oxygen can be supplied with a portable, lightweight cylinder, and short-burst (SBOT) and long-term (LTOT) oxygen therapy supplied from an oxygen concentrator. Nasal cannulae are usually better tolerated than a mask, but the latter is necessary when controlled oxygen delivery (e.g. 24%) is required. See 📚 Chapter 5, pp. 76–77 for further details.

Parenteral drug infusions

If a patient is unable to take oral medications, drugs may be given using the subcutaneous route. A continuous subcutaneous infusion of medications such as opioids, anxiolytics, and anti-emetics can provide good symptom control in the home. Potential drugs and doses are described in Table 12.4 pp. 258–259. Syringe drivers are small, light, battery-operated, and easily portable in a cloth bag carried on the shoulder or around the neck. Only once-daily visits from the healthcare team are needed to refill the syringe driver.

Non-invasive ventilation

Nocturnal NIV, using a portable non-invasive positive pressure ventilator, is feasible and easily used at home, particularly for patients with neuro-muscular causes of respiratory failure such as motor neurone disease. A nasal mask is usually best tolerated, often with the addition of a humidifier. See 📚 Chapter 2, pp. 40–42 for further details.

Chapter 12

Care in the terminal phase

Introduction

'The ultimate challenge for us is to accompany them as far as we can on that journey that one day we too must make.'

Fürst and Doyle, 2005

The terminal phase is defined as being when a patient enters the last few days or hours of life. Terminal care is not simply a replication of the care given over the preceding weeks. New problems commonly arise that must be proactively sought out and addressed. It is tragic for a patient who has had high quality care during their illness to die suffering in body or mind. The memory of such distress is never forgotten by relatives and can over-ride other good memories, compounding their grief.

Diagnosing dying

The last days or hours of life are characterized by a number of features:
- profound weakness
- increasing drowsiness
- difficulty concentrating and sometimes confusion
- reducing intake of fluid and food
- difficulty swallowing medication
- increasing time in bed and dependence on help.

Diagnosing dying can be challenging for a number of reasons:
- Many, if not all, of the above features may not be new.
- Reversible causes of deterioration, such as infection, may cause similar features.

In practice, a patient with advanced disease is likely to be entering the terminal phase when:
- the above features have been developing over many days or weeks
- reversible causes of deterioration have been excluded
- the deterioration in condition is worsening day by day.

Goals of care

A number of principles of a good death have been identified:[1,2]
- To know when death is coming and to understand what can be expected.
- To retain control over what happens, including decision-making about treatment, place of death, and control over who is present.
- To have time for completion, including individual life review, resolution of conflicts, spending time with family and friends, making plans for after death (such as funeral arrangements), and saying goodbye.
- To be afforded dignity and privacy, with affirmation of the whole person.
- To have access to good pain relief and other symptom control, and to emotional and spiritual support.

Few of these principles are achievable without recognition that death is relatively imminent. Therefore, despite the inherent challenges, it is of vital importance that dying is recognized, in order that appropriate and compassionate care can be provided.

References

1. Debate of the Age, Health and Care Study Group (1999) *The Future of Health and Care of Older People: The best is yet to come*. Age Concern, London.
2. Steinhauser KE, Clipp EC, McNeilly M et al. (2000) In search of a good death: observations of patients, families, and providers. *Ann Intern Med*, 132: 825–832.

Domains of care in the terminal phase

Physical

Patients tend to suffer from a range of physical symptoms in the terminal phase, with symptoms both emerging for the first time and recurring. The majority of patients with advanced respiratory disease will experience to some extent fatigue, anorexia, breathlessness, and a dry mouth. Many will also suffer from restlessness or agitation, noisy breathing with excess secretions, and pain.

Drowsy or confused patients may not be able to communicate the existence of uncontrolled symptoms. Therefore, proactive assessment of the risk of specific symptoms must be made, based on knowledge of the underlying pathological process. Non-verbal cues and other evidence from examination are helpful.

There is evidence to suggest that relatives suspect patients are experiencing more symptoms than may actually be occurring. Anxious relatives may, for example, interpret grunting or restlessness as evidence of pain. Clinical assessment for the presence of symptoms must, nevertheless, be undertaken before careful explanation and reassurance can be given.

Detailed guidelines for the management of specific symptoms in the terminal phase are given on 📖 pp. 246–250.

Psychospiritual

The majority of patients entering the terminal phase appear to be aware of how ill they are and that they are likely to die soon. However, relatives tend to be less aware than the patient. Even if they suspect the prognosis is short, they may not act in accordance with this, so as to 'protect' the patient from the truth. This, combined with the fact that healthcare professionals may still be talking about further tests and treatment, can lead to confusion and exacerbate anxiety in both patients and their families.

When approaching death, people usually look both forwards and backwards. Looking ahead, it is common to fear the process of dying more than the prospect of being dead. Those who can articulate their thoughts speak of the following:

- Fear of future suffering, and of uncontrolled symptoms such as pain.
- Concern about being subjected to further investigations and interventions such as enemata.
- Dread of dying 'struggling for breath', 'choking to death', 'suffocating', or alone.
- Concern about being a 'burden' on their family.
- Sadness about never seeing their loved ones again.
- Anxiety as to how family members will cope during the dying process and after death.
- Fear of going to sleep in case they never wake up again.

The terminal phase is also a time when people look back, reviewing life.
- Trying to make sense of both what has happened during their past lives and what is happening now.
- Attempting to judge the 'usefulness' of their life.

- Trying to understand the meaning of life and of suffering.
- Regretting past conflicts and disputes and desiring reconciliation and forgiveness.

Patients who believe in a religion may frame such questions and answers within the context of their faith. On occasion, doubts about long-standing religious beliefs may be expressed at this stage.

Patients will choose when and with whom to discuss their concerns. Thoughts may be articulated at unexpected moments, such as when being washed. Articulating fears can be cathartic. Compassionate listening is the greatest way of helping, without comment or judgement, simply 'being alongside', easing the loneliness of the patient's journey.

Social

Relatives suffer in many ways during and after the terminal phase of a patient's illness. They may not be able to accept or understand that the patient is dying. This may be reflected in energetic encouragement of feeding, hydration, or medical intervention.

Many factors contribute to the almost inevitable sense of fear. In societies where the majority of people die in hospital, relatives may have had little personal experience of death and dying. The 'unknown' is, by definition, frightening, including both uncertainties relating to the timing and nature of dying, and the prospect of coping without the family member in the future.

By encouraging and giving time for open communication, healthcare professionals can provide invaluable support for relatives and carers. This may also benefit the patient, who may be relieved to know that loved ones are receiving help.

Practical measures can support patients and their relatives. For example, social workers or appropriate agencies may be able to help with concerns relating to financial matters or dependent relatives. The social domain of care must never be overlooked. Addressing these issues can resolve distress and contribute to life coming to a peaceful end.

Preparation for death

'Despair is most often the offspring of ill-preparedness.'

Don Williams Jr

Proactive preparation for death is of great importance and can have an immeasurable impact on the terminal phase and its aftermath.

Once it has become apparent that a patient is dying, there are usually a large number of matters that need to be addressed. High quality care prior to the terminal phase should mean that some aspects of preparation have already occurred. Checklists can be useful at this stage, including that provided in the initial assessment of the Liverpool Care Pathway for the Dying Patient (see 📖 Chapter 11, pp. 234–235).

Communication

- Is the patient aware that he/she is dying? Some patients choose to talk about this explicitly. A significant proportion acknowledge their impending death implicitly: 'I know I'm not well…' or 'Please look out for my wife…' Be observant for cues.
- Are relatives aware that the patient is dying? This usually needs to be discussed explicitly, with care and compassion. Uncertainty or imagined outcomes may be more frightening than the truth.
- Have the patient and relatives or carers been given time to discuss any matters that are of importance to them, including hopes, fears, and wishes? Have decisions been made about the place of death and those chosen to provide care and support? Table 12.1 outlines potential advantages and disadvantages of three places of death.
- Has the patient's GP or other key healthcare professional been notified? Are professionals that can provide specialist support available if necessary, such as a chaplain, social worker, or family support worker?
- Are contact details available for the next of kin and other important contacts? Have attempts been made to optimize communication with the patient and relatives, for example using hearing aids or interpreters? Have information leaflets been given if appropriate?
- Has advice been given to relatives about calling distant family and friends, particularly those that have the greatest distance to travel?
- If a post mortem is likely to be mandatory (for example in diseases where financial compensation may be considered, such as mesothelioma), has the next of kin been warned of this likelihood?
- Have patients or relatives been given the opportunity to express wishes in relation to tissue donation (such as corneas, skin, bone) after death?

Medical intervention

- Has a review of all medications been taken, identifying those that can be discontinued (see Table 12.2)? If the oral route becomes unavailable, through which route will medications be given?
- Has the patient been prescribed on an 'as needed' basis any medications that may be required to control symptoms? Are all such

medications available? Who will administer these drugs?
(See p. 260).
- For patients in hospital, has a decision been made in relation to further monitoring (blood glucose, vital signs, oxygen saturation) or investigations (blood tests, chest X-ray)?
- Has a decision been made not to attempt cardiopulmonary resuscitation? Is the outcome of this decision available to all who need it, including out of hours and emergency ambulance services? If the patient has an implanted defibrillator, has this been deactivated?
- Have decisions been made about whether artificial hydration will be given? A reduced need for fluids (and food) is part of the dying process, and clinically assisted hydration is rarely necessary. Good mouth care usually alleviates thirst/dry mouth more than hydration (see p. 252).
- For patients using non-invasive ventilation (NIV), whether to improve survival or palliate breathlessness, has a decision been made about whether or not to continue it? If it is to be discontinued, is a withdrawal plan in place (see p. 262–263)?
- Has the patient's skin integrity been assessed? Has a recognized risk assessment tool been used to support clinical judgement? Has the frequency of repositioning been determined?
- What method will be used if the patient does not have a catheter and is no longer able to pass urine in a bedpan or bottle? Are pads, catheter, or convene appropriate?

Equipment

- Is equipment available to support a continuous subcutaneous infusion of medication?
- If the patient is at home, is he or she on an appropriate mattress or in a hospital bed? Are all potentially useful nursing aids available?
- Is a portable (but not necessarily hand-held) fan available to palliate breathlessness? If NIV is to be continued for symptom control, is the equipment available?

Table 12.1 Preferred place of care

	Potential advantages	Potential disadvantages
Home	Familiar and cherished setting. Relaxed, peaceful and non-medical atmosphere. Care from familiar primary healthcare team. No need for family to travel to visit patient. Family may sleep better in their own beds.	Lack of 24 hour nursing care. Increased risk of a sense of isolation or fear. Lack of equipment and necessary drugs. Out of hours medical support may not know the patient. Not necessarily 24hr access to palliative care advice. Potentially excessive visitors and phone calls.
Acute hospital	Patient may be well known to the team. 24 hour access to nurses, doctors and drugs. Security of knowing there will be support in a crisis. Possibility of acute intervention to relieve symptoms eg drainage of pleural effusion.	Potentially noisy, particularly at night. Lack of private space for patient and family. Not necessarily 24hr access to palliative care advice. Acute care, inappropriate investigation or intervention. Implicit sense of 'medical failure.' Exhausting for family to visit, and limit of visitors allowed.
Hospice setting	More peaceful and 'home like' than hospital setting. Unlimited visiting, and usually space for family to stay. 24 hour access to nurses, doctors and drugs. Specialist palliative care expertise in complex situations. Atmosphere of acceptance of death and making the best of remaining life.	Insufficient beds for all dying patients, traditional focus on patients with cancer. Patients or relatives not accepting of impending death may become frightened or depressed. May be far for family to travel.

Table 12.2 Review of drugs in the terminal phase

Continue (or start 'as needed')	Consider stopping	Stop
Analgesics (pain)	Antiarrhythmics	Antihypertensives
Antiemetics (nausea, vomiting)	Diuretics	Cholesterol-lowering drugs
Anxiolytics (anxiety, dyspnoea)	Oral hypoglycaemics[a]	Laxatives
Sedatives (agitation)	Anticonvulsants	Gastroprotection
Antimuscarinics (secretions)	Steroids[b]	Prophylactic antibiotics
	Antidepressants	Dietary supplements
		Anticoagulation

a: Consider monitoring glucose occasionally

b: Unless high dose for more than a week, controlling symptoms from raised intracranial pressure, or long term use for co-morbidity

Management of breathlessness

Control of breathlessness in the terminal phase moves from predominantly non-pharmacological to pharmacological measures. The aim of treatment is to alleviate the perception of breathlessness and associated anxiety.

Three classes of drugs can be used (see 📖 Chapter 5, pp. 78–80):
- Opioids: reduce the perception of breathlessness.
- Benzodiazepines: relieve anxiety.
- Antipsychotics: relieve extreme anxiety and agitation.

These drugs are usually given through the subcutaneous route, if or when the oral route becomes unavailable. Benzodiazepines can also have a rapid onset of action when given through the sublingual route e.g. lorazepam 0.5mg sublingual bd prn.

There is rarely a role for oxygen in the terminal phase. Psychological dependence on oxygen may have occurred, however, requiring careful explanation before gradual withdrawal.

Clinical tips:
- A continuous subcutaneous infusion (CSCI) of both low-dose morphine (or diamorphine) and low-dose midazolam is recommended as an effective method for palliating breathlessness at the very end of life.
- If opioid naïve, commence morphine sulphate 5–10mg with midazolam 5–10mg CSCI over 24 hours, and titrate according to response.
- If already on opioids, convert to parenteral route and consider small dose increase with further upward titration as needed.

Mr G was a 78-year-old man with end-stage COPD. He required hospital admission every few weeks for exacerbations of breathlessness. In recent weeks he had become entirely bed-bound. Following extensive care planning discussions, he and his family decided that he would stay at home the next time he developed a chest infection, using oral antibiotics without escalation. He gained reasonable symptom control using morphine sulphate immediate release 1.5mg six hourly, and lorazepam 0.5mg sublingually at times of acute breathlessness. His GP had recently converted him to morphine sulphate modified release 5mg bd po.

After a severe infection that did not respond significantly to oral antibiotics, it became apparent that Mr G was now entering the terminal phase of his illness. He was converted to a CSCI containing morphine sulphate 10mg and midazolam 10mg, the syringe driver being refilled every 24 hours by his district nurse. Although his breathlessness was reasonably controlled initially, he then started to become restless, with agitation and disorientation at night. Haloperidol 5mg was added to the infusion with good effect. He died the next day, following a peaceful night.

Management of retained secretions

Patients in the terminal phase tend to be too weak to clear or expectorate respiratory tract secretions. This can lead to noisy respiration, a condition known as 'death rattle'. This common symptom occurs in up to 90% of patients dying of all causes, and is almost ubiquitous in patients with advanced respiratory disease.

The sound of noisy respiration with excess secretions is distressing for relatives and health carers. It is believed, however, that this symptom does not particularly distress patients, who tend at this stage to be either semiconscious or unconscious.

Undertaking research in vulnerable and potentially unconscious patients is fraught with difficulty, and there is no placebo-controlled trial evidence to support any intervention for this condition.

Despite this, the following interventions are commonly used:

- Change of lying position to semi-prone position to encourage postural drainage.
- Parenteral anti-secretory drugs: glycopyrronium, hyoscine butylbromide, hyoscine hydrobromide (see Table 12.4 for drug details).

There is anecdotal and uncontrolled trial experience that anti-secretory drugs reduce the noise of 'death rattle'. It is not known whether or not they impact on the patient's quality of life. The drugs can, however, have adverse effects including uncomfortable thickening of secretions and dry mouth. Hyoscine hydrobromide crosses the blood-brain barrier and can cause sedation and, occasionally, paradoxical agitation.

Clinical tips:
- Reassure relatives that this type of noisy breathing is not believed to be distressing for patients.
- Try moving the patient to a semi-prone position.
- Avoid using anti-muscarinic drugs if possible.

Management of pain

The presence of pain is under-recognized in patients with advanced respiratory disease, particularly in those with non-malignant disease. Detailed information on pain management is given in Chapter 6.

In the dying patient, a high suspicion for the presence of pain should be maintained. As well as malignant pain, musculoskeletal pain from chest wall or immobility is relatively common in this phase. As always, reversible causes of pain or discomfort should be considered, including pressure sores, urinary retention, and constipation.

If the oral route is not available, the following options can be considered:

- Opioid analgesia can be given by continuous subcutaneous infusion. For example, a patient on codeine phosphate 60mg qds could be converted to morphine sulphate 10mg/24hrs CSCI with 1.5–2.5mg sc prn for breakthrough pain.
- Sublingual fentanyl tablets can relieve short-lived or incident pain in patients already on at least 60mg/24hrs oral morphine sulphate (see 📖 p. 107). The starting dose is 100mcg, irrespective of the background opioid dose, and this can be titrated up to a maximum of 800mcg per dose.
- NSAIDs are particularly effective for musculoskeletal and pleuritic pain, and can be given per rectum if the oral route is unavailable. For severe pain, ketorolac can be given by CSCI.
- Agents for neuropathic pain, such as amitriptyline and gabapentin, cannot be given parenterally. Parenteral options include use of methadone and ketamine. Although, in practice, these drugs rarely need to be commenced in the terminal phase, if necessary they can be used with advice from a specialist palliative care team.

Clinical tips:

- Have a low threshold for considering the presence of pain, including in patients with non-malignant localized respiratory disease.
- Low-dose opioid infusion can palliate both pain and breathlessness.

Management of agitation

Restlessness and agitation are unfortunately relatively common symptoms in the terminal phase, occurring to some degree in up to 40% of patients. It is important to deal with such problems actively as, unchecked, the negative impact on both the patient's dignity and on relatives' last memories of the deceased can be devastating.

Causes

There are a large number of potential causes of agitation in the terminal phase. Distress from pain, nausea, urinary retention, and constipation, as well as fear and anxiety, can all cause restlessness or even agitation.

Agitation, particularly when associated with confusion and/or drowsiness, may be a symptom of an acute organic brain syndrome or delirium. This is sometimes termed a 'terminal agitation', but arguably should more accurately be called a 'terminal delirium'. Causes of terminal delirium include the following:

- drugs
- biochemical derangement
- infection
- cerebral hypoxia.

A large number of drugs can cause agitation, including anti-muscarinic drugs and steroids. Even benzodiazepines can cause a paradoxical agitation in some patients because of their disorientating effect. Drug levels may be increased by reduction in renal or hepatic clearance, exacerbating the problem. Iatrogenic agitation can usually easily be reversed by stopping or reducing the dose of the drug.

Other causes of delirium in the terminal phase may be less easy or inappropriate to attempt to correct, including biochemical derangement (e.g. hyponatraemia) or infection.

Management

Once reversible causes that are appropriate and feasible to treat have been corrected, the mainstay of management is pharmacological. Midazolam, haloperidol, and levomepromazine are useful, as they can easily be given by subcutaneous infusion (see Table 12.4 for drug details). Haloperidol and levomepromazine both have an anti-emetic effect, particularly for biochemical causes of nausea, which may be of value in patients with a terminal biochemical disturbance or opioid-induced nausea.

Non-drug approaches are also of significant value, including the presence of a close relative, continuity of carers, and a safe and peaceful environment.

> *Clinical tips:*
> - Always consider drug-induced agitation or confusion.
> - A continuous subcutaneous infusion (CSCI) of midazolam can palliate both agitation and breathlessness.
> - Haloperidol CSCI can palliate agitation, confusion, hiccups, and opioid- or drug-induced nausea.

General comfort measures

Other symptoms

Nausea and vomiting

Nausea is prevalent in the terminal phase. The commonest causes and first choice of anti-emetic are detailed in Table 12.3. The rationale for anti-emetic choice is described on see 📖 pp. 134–136.

- Always use the subcutaneous route for anti-emetic administration.
- If the first-line anti-emetic is not effective, change to levomepromazine. As well as being effective for a range of causes, this drug can reduce anxiety and, at higher doses, cause a degree of sedation.

Dry mouth

This symptom is almost ubiquitous in patients with advanced respiratory disease in the terminal phase. A rapid respiratory rate and mouth breathing lead to evaporation of fluid from the mouth. Use of an oxygen mask compounds the problem and, as described earlier, is not recommended.

- Treat reversible causes, such as by stopping anti-muscarinic drugs and treating oral candidiasis (if able to use antifungal medication, such as nystatin).
- Provide good mouth care, debriding a furred tongue with a soft toothbrush or placing a ¼ ascorbic acid tablet on the tongue.
- Smear paraffin ointment on the lips.
- Encourage regular sips of cold water or carbonated lemonade, or sucking of ice chips.
- Consider regular use of artificial saliva sprays (e.g. Saliva Orthana®).

Cough

Unlike at earlier stages, in the terminal phase cough suppression is usually necessary, irrespective of whether the cough is wet or dry.

- In patients no longer able to swallow, if opioid naïve start a low-dose morphine sulphate infusion (5–10mg/24hrs CSCI, titrating up to effect).
- Patients already receiving opioids may require a dose increase.

Haemoptysis

Patients with advanced respiratory disease are at risk of haemoptysis. A large volume haemoptysis can be extremely distressing for patients, carers, and staff.

- Have a red or green blanket easily available to disguise the volume of blood loss.
- Consider use of large-bolus doses of midazolam (e.g. 5–10mg sc stat) or levomepromazine (e.g. 12.5–25mg sc stat), as well as strong opioids.
- If at home, consider using sublingual lorazepam (1mg) or buccal midazolam (2.5–10mg).

Skin care

Skin integrity

Patients in the terminal phase are at high risk of pressure sores and loss of skin integrity, particularly those that are taking steroids.

- Regular nursing skin assessment and repositioning is important. The frequency of this should be tailored to the needs of each individual patient.

Hygiene

Personal hygiene continues to be of great importance during the terminal phase. Body odour can be distressing, particularly to close relatives.

- Gentle cleaning of eyes, face, and sweaty areas of skin can be refreshing and improve comfort significantly.
- Changes of clothes may be needed, particularly if a patient has been sweating excessively.
- Some family members may find it comforting to be involved in providing this personal care.

Hydration and nutrition

Fluids

A degree of dehydration is part of the normal dying process. Full hydration can lead to peripheral or sacral oedema, pulmonary oedema, or cerebral oedema, as capillary oncotic pressures fall and fluid moves across damaged membranes.

- Patients may choose to take sips of cold drinks. Relatives may enjoy being able to help the patient with this. Closer to death, hot drinks tend to become less enjoyable.
- There is rarely a need for parenteral fluids in the last days of life. Hydration can cause harm as described above. Relatives invariably understand and accept the situation when this is explained compassionately.
- Moist mucous membranes in the mouth can alleviate the feeling of thirst. Good mouth care, rather than forced hydration, is the key.

Food

Appetite decreases as death approaches, which can cause great distress to relatives. There is no evidence to suggest that artificial enteral or parenteral nutrition contribute to comfort and, indeed, such measures may cause nausea, abdominal bloating, or discomfort.

- Offer patients tiny mouthfuls of any food they fancy. Relatives may enjoy helping with feeding, as well as sourcing the chosen food.
- Stop corticosteroids or progestogens that were started to improve anorexia.
- Careful explanation for relatives is vital, including describing the potential discomfort caused by unwanted food and the likely fact that the food will not be metabolized or 'turned into useful energy'.

Bladder and bowel

Distress associated with the need to micturate or defaecate, or the consequences of incontinence, can contribute to agitation in the terminal phase.

- Most patients in the terminal phase will either require incontinence pads or urethral catheterization.
- Bowel intervention may not be needed unless there is evidence that a patient is experiencing discomfort. Gentle rectal measures, such as a glycerin suppository, may be all that is needed.

Psychological care

Attention to the patient's psychological well-being remains of great importance during the last days and hours of life.

- Be available to listen or respond to questions or concerns. Sitting quietly at the bedside can be a great support, particularly if there are no relatives present.
- Consider spiritual and cultural needs carefully, involving appropriate professionals, if needed, as well as relatives.

Environment

The environment of the place of death needs to be adjusted to the specific needs of each patient.

- Sufficient space by the bedside, privacy, and a calm atmosphere are usually valued. A call bell needs to be accessible.
- Consider use of fragrance, silence, or music. Relatives may be prompted to consider bringing photographs.

Carer needs

Carers tend to feel helpless, sad, and fearful. Physical exhaustion after a long illness can compound their emotional turmoil. They often focus on the needs of the patient, to the detriment of their own.

- Healthcare professionals should encourage carers to consider their own needs, including drinking, eating, and taking periods of rest.
- It is important to be available to answer questions and provide explanations. Relatives may gain comfort from knowing that a patient may be able to hear them, even when not responding.
- If families wish children or grandchildren to visit, it is important that they explain to the child what the patient will look like and whether they will be able to speak. Children should be encouraged to talk about the visit afterwards.

Table 12.3 First-line antiemetics in the terminal phase

Cause	Examples	First line antiemetic
Biochemical derangement	Renal impairment, respiratory acidosis, hypercalcaemia	Haloperidol 2.5-5mg/24hrs CSCI
Drug accumulation	Opioid accumulation in renal impairment	Haloperidol 2.5-5mg/24hrs CSCI
Raised intracranial pressure	Small cell lung cancer with brain metastases	Cyclizine 100-150mg/24hrs CSCI
Gastric stasis	Immobility	Metoclopramide 30-60mg/24hrs CSCI

Syringe drivers

A continuous subcutaneous infusion (CSCI) using a syringe driver (SD) is an effective form of drug delivery when the oral route is not available. The advantages are as follows:

- An infusion is more comfortable than repeated injections.
- There is maintenance of steady plasma drug concentrations without peaks and troughs, so improving symptom control.
- A number of drugs can be combined, controlling a range of symptoms with one infusion.
- The driver is lightweight and portable, avoiding hindering mobility.
- The syringe only needs to be refilled once daily, which can occur in the community, as well as inpatient settings.

A syringe driver may be indicated when a patient is unable to take oral medication, for reasons that include the following:

- weakness or drowsiness in the terminal phase
- nausea and vomiting
- dysphagia
- bowel obstruction
- severe malabsorption.

Practical points

Drug doses

Table 12.4 outlines usual doses for the most commonly used drugs. Note that drugs with a longer half-life or duration of action, such as dexamethasone and levomepromazine, can if necessary be administered as a single bolus subcutaneous injection rather than a continuous infusion.

Drugs are generally more bioavailable when given parenterally than orally. This gives an approximate guide to dose reduction when converting from the oral to subcutaneous route. For example, the dose of a 50% bioavailable oral drug can be approximately halved when given parenterally.

Drug compatibility

Up to three and, on occasion, four drugs can be administered together in a syringe. The majority of the commonly used drugs are compatible with each other. Care is needed when cyclizine is combined with higher doses of opioids, and when using dexamethasone. The stability of drug combinations can be increased by the following:

- Dilute to the maximum volume.
- Deliver over no more than 24 hours.
- Protect from direct sunlight (especially if containing levomepromazine).
- Avoid higher temperatures, keeping above bed covers if possible.

Useful information on drug compatibility is available on:

- www.palliativedrugs.com
- www.pallcare.info

Diluent

Water for injection (WFI) or 0.9% saline can be used. WFI is most widely used in the UK because of the increased compatibility data available, and the increased chance of compatibility with cyclizine. There is, however, more data to support dilution of octreotide and ketamine in saline.

Timing of starting

Start the syringe driver 1–2 hours before the oral form of the medication is due to wear off. If symptoms are poorly controlled, give bolus doses (see Table 12.4) and start the SD at the same time.

A 72-year-old man with small cell lung cancer and brain metastases was becoming increasingly drowsy, and it was clear that his prognosis was measured in hours or short days. He became unable to take his oral medications, morphine sulphate MR 50mg bd, cyclizine 50mg tds, and dexamethasone 4mg bd.

He was converted to a SD containing morphine sulphate 50mg and cyclizine 150mg. This was commenced at 19.00, 10 hours after his last oral morphine sulphate dose. As a recent increase in dexamethasone dose had been highly effective in alleviating severe headaches, he was also commenced on daily subcutaneous dexamethasone injections, 6mg each morning (oral bioavailability ~80%).

Setting up

- Preferred sites for infusion are the anterior chest, abdomen, and thighs, and the anterolateral aspects of the upper arms. Avoid skin folds, bony prominences, and oedematous areas.
- Follow the instructions for the particular SD device being used, and set a rate so that the medication is delivered over a 24-hour period (mL/24hrs or mm/24hrs).
- Check that the battery is sufficiently charged, and recheck the driver at a maximum of 4-hourly intervals to monitor the skin site and check that the infusion is running to time.

Troubleshooting

Infusion site reactions

Local site reactions are most likely to occur if the site is older than 72 hours or the SD contains cyclizine, levomepromazine, or high doses of diamorphine. A number of steps can be taken to try to prevent reactions:

- Dilute the solution as much as feasible (20mL or 30mL syringe).
- Rotate the site every 72 hours.
- Change the drug combination.
- If adequate compatibility data, use 0.9% saline instead of WFI.

Use of low-dose dexamethasone has been advocated but, in practice, can lead to drug incompatibility issues.

Syringe driver unavailable

- Use another pump, such as those used for intravenous infusions, as an interim measure.
- Use bolus doses of the drugs at regular intervals, aiming if possible to prescribe drugs with a longer duration of action on a once daily basis (e.g. levomepromazine).

Table 12.4 Drugs for subcutaneous infusion in the terminal phase

Drug	Role/indications	Dose CSCI/24hrs	Bolus dose 'prn'	Comments
Alfentanil	Pain (in renal failure) Breathlessness	0.5–1mg (or 1/10 of the 24hr diamorphine dose)	1/6–1/8 of the 24hr dose	Involve specialist palliative care colleagues if unfamiliar with this drug. Less evidence to support its use in breathlessness than for morphine. Very short half-life, so bolus doses short-acting.
Cyclizine	N+V (raised intracranial pressure, vertigo)	100–150mg	50mg	Can be sedating and causes dry mouth. Risk of incompatibility with high-dose diamorphine. Can cause site reactions. Never combine with metoclopramide. Combines well with haloperidol.
Dexamethasone	Raised intracranial pressure Anti-emetic	4–12mg	-	Can give as single sc dose, as long duration of action. Give in morning to avoid nocturnal sleep disturbance or agitation.
Diamorphine	Pain Breathlessness Cough	Start at 5–10mg if opioid naive	2.5mg if opioid naive	Effective for breathlessness in combination with midazolam. Three times as potent as oral morphine.
Glycopyrronium	Excess secretions	0.6–1.2mg	0.2mg	Causes dry mouth. Can make secretions sticky and more distressing. No central adverse effects as does not cross blood-brain barrier.
Haloperidol	N+V (chemical causes e.g. renal failure) Anxiety/delirium Hiccups	2.5–5.0mg	1.5–2.5mg	Valuable drug because of range of actions, and likelihood of chemical causes of nausea in the terminal phase (drug accumulation, renal/hepatic impairment etc.).

Hyoscine butylbromide	Excess secretions Abdominal colic	40mg (secretions) 60mg (colic)	20mg	Causes dry mouth. Can make secretions sticky and more distressing.
Hyoscine hydrobromide	Excess secretions	1.2–2.4mg	0.4mg	Useful in the terminal phase when sedation also required. Risk of paradoxical agitation. Can be administered by topical route (Scopoderm® patch).
Levomepromazine	N+V (broad spectrum) Distress/anxiety/delirium Insomnia	12.5–100mg	6.25–12.5mg	Valuable drug because of wide range of actions. Very sedating in higher doses. Helpful in severe terminal agitation/ delirium. Long duration of action means can be given as once daily sc injection instead of CSCI.
Metoclopramide	N+V (functional bowel obstruction, gastric stasis)	30–90mg	10mg	Continue in the terminal phase if already in use and effective. Do not combine with cyclizine or levomepromazine.
Morphine sulphate	Pain Breathlessness Cough	Start at 10mg if opioid naïve	2.5mg–5mg if opioid naïve	Effective for breathlessness in combination with midazolam. Twice as potent as oral morphine.
Midazolam	Distress/anxiety Breathlessness Insomnia	10–100mg	2.5–10mg	Particular role for breathlessness in the terminal phase, as breathlessness always associated with anxiety. Bolus doses can potentially be given through the buccal route for acute breathlessness, if stat sc doses not immediately available— unlicensed.

Anticipatory prescribing

It is vital to anticipate symptoms that may occur in the terminal phase in order to ensure prompt and effective symptom control. Anticipatory prescribing is an important step in facilitating patient comfort in the terminal phase.

- Prescribe appropriate drugs to be given as subcutaneous bolus injections on an 'as required' basis.
- Make sure the drugs are available, including creating a store in the patient's own home if necessary.

The following types of drugs should be prescribed. Bolus dose sizes are contained in Table 12.4:

- analgesic e.g. morphine sulphate
- anti-emetic e.g. usual anti-emetic, haloperidol, or levomepromazine
- anxiolytic e.g. midazolam, haloperidol
- anti-secretory agent e.g. hyoscine butylbromide, glycopyrronium.

Haloperidol, midazolam, and morphine are particularly valuable because of their ability to alleviate a number of symptoms each.

Withdrawal of ventilation

A number of scenarios can arise in patients with advanced respiratory disease who are receiving non-invasive ventilation (NIV) or invasive ventilation as they approach the end of life:

- A patient experiences progressive symptoms despite use of NIV, and chooses either to continue or, less commonly, to withdraw the NIV during the last days of life.
- An intubated patient is making no progress or is deteriorating. Ventilation is withdrawn because continued treatment would be futile, and there is little prospect of surviving without ventilation.

Patients in these scenarios are likely to have limited capacity to make these important decisions at the time. Careful advance care planning is therefore vital (see 📖 Chapter 8, pp. 174–176). Any patient commenced on NIV should be involved in discussion about potential discontinuation, before NIV is commenced.

A decision as to whether withdrawal of ventilation is in the best interests of a patient without capacity should take into account medical information, any statement of wishes and preferences, and the views of relatives. A valid advance decision may determine the decision to be taken. The ethical aspects of decision-making in this context are described in Chapter 9.

Preparation

Careful preparation is the key to successful withdrawal of ventilation. An explicit plan with a checklist can ensure that every step is attended to and no details are forgotten.

Once the decision to withdraw ventilation has been made, a number of steps need to be taken.

Communication with family

- Describe the likely outcome of withdrawal of ventilation, including the types of respiratory pattern that may precede death.
- Discuss the possibility that death may not occur rapidly and, if appropriate, touch on potential plans for future management.
- Explain the process of ventilation withdrawal, including the rationale for stopping monitoring.
- If appropriate and necessary, sensitively discuss the possibility of a post mortem or of organ or tissue donation.
- Agree on the timing of withdrawal of ventilation.

Initial preparation

- Inform appropriate members of the wider multidisciplinary team, including, for example, a chaplain, social worker, or tissue donation coordinator.
- Try to create a quiet and relatively private space for the patient and family. With care, this is usually possible even in an intensive care unit setting.

- Decide on who will perform the withdrawal, and the method of withdrawal.
- Discontinue investigations and treatments that are not needed for comfort, such as antibiotics.
- Wean off neuromuscular blocking agents and ensure the patient is comfortable with the use of appropriate analgesic and anxiolytic medication.

Final preparation

- Stop and, where possible, remove monitoring equipment.
- Ensure that drugs that can relieve respiratory distress (opioids and benzodiazepines) are available and, in some instances, already drawn up to facilitate rapid parenteral delivery. Patients already receiving these drugs may require extra bolus doses.
- Check that suction equipment is available and ready to use.

Withdrawal

There is no established optimal method of withdrawal of ventilation. Prolonged 'terminal weaning' may increase the distress of the patient and/or family by prolonging the dying process. On the other hand, abrupt discontinuation of ventilatory support may cause sudden onset of dyspnoea or distress. In practice, an approach between these extremes may be best. A deliberate graded reduction of the ventilator pressure settings over several hours can be combined with administration of opioids and benzodiazepines, titrated according to the patient's changing clinical condition.

Non-invasive ventilation

Many patients choose to continue NIV during the last days of life, despite progressive symptoms and the noise and slight discomfort inherent in NIV use. However, with reassurance that potential symptoms can be controlled pharmacologically, it is usually possible to remove the NIV rather earlier. This can improve the comfort and peacefulness of the terminal phase.

Invasive ventilation

It is considered best practice to remove the endotracheal tube at some point once the ventilator settings have been weaned. The tube left in place can contribute to discomfort, medicalizes the dying process, and can leave lasting memories for family of disfigurement of the patient's face. It can be a source of great comfort to family members to be able to see and kiss a face that is free from medical equipment.

Further reading

Dickman A, Schneider J, Varga J (2005) *The Syringe Driver: Continuous subcutaneous infusions in palliative care*, 2ⁿᵈ edition. Oxford University Press, Oxford.

Fürst C, Doyle D (2005) The terminal phase. In: Doyle D, Hanks G, Cherny N, Calman K (eds.), *Oxford Textbook of Palliative Medicine*, 3ʳᵈ edition. Oxford University Press, Oxford, pp1117–1134.

Royal College of Physicians, British Thoracic Society, Intensive Care Society (2008) *Non-invasive Ventilation in Chronic Obstructive Pulmonary Disease: Management of acute type 2 respiratory failure*. Concise Guidance to Good Practice series, No. 11. RCP, London.

Truog R, Campbell M, Randall Curtis J, *et al.* (2008) Recommendations for end of life care in the intensive care unit: a consensus statement by the American College of Critical Care Medicine. *Crit Care Med*; 36 (3): 953–963.

Chapter 13

Spiritual and cultural needs

Introduction

'Death is like a mirror in which the true meaning of life is reflected.'

Sogyal Rinpoche

'Real spirituality is all about what you do with your pain—you either transmit it or transform it!'

Richard Rohr

This chapter is concerned with helping those dying with advanced, chronic respiratory disease to have access to spiritual and culturally sensitive care. High quality end of life care encompasses working effectively with patients' and families' beliefs and philosophical orientation, as well as the provision of clinical care.

In no other period of a person's life can spirituality and philosophy, in their broadest senses, mean so much, influencing equanimity and often having an impact on symptom control.

Importance of addressing spiritual and cultural needs

'It is much more important to know what sort of a patient has a disease, than what sort of disease a patient has.'

Sir William Osler

Most societies in the West are now multicultural to some degree. Understanding cultural diversity is now a feature of undergraduate and post-graduate professional development, with provision of 'diversity training'. Increasing priority is being given to cultural and spiritual aspects of care because they affect access to and use of services, and the quality of care given, particularly to the dying.

Accessing services

It is increasingly recognized that patients from ethnic minorities and from poorer sections of society:

- receive a lower standard of healthcare in general
- are less likely to use specialist palliative care services.

Some of the underuse of health services may relate to invisible, 'unthinking' barriers to access, services having been designed to fit the needs of the dominant culture. In addition, as the West becomes increasingly secular, in contrast to some of the ethnic communities, the importance of religion may be underestimated.

Hospices can be perceived as forbidding places by patients from ethnic minorities. They may even feel that they are places that accelerate or accentuate death, where a person will be required to give up hope in order to be admitted. The Christian ethos of some hospices may also be a barrier to those of a non-Christian faith. Such perceptions can prevent those who would otherwise greatly benefit from hospice care from receiving it.

Table 13.1 Religion versus spirituality *(Max Watson; unpublished work)*

Religion	Spirituality
From Latin *religio*, to rebind	From Latin *spiritus*, breathing
System of practices and beliefs	Dynamic process
Influenced by social, historical and cultural factors	Gives existential meaning to life events
Community	Individual
The *map*	The *journey*

Controlling symptoms

Cicely Saunders described 'total pain' as pain with social, psychological, and spiritual aspects, as well as physical ones. Her ideas are now encompassed in the 'bio-psychosocial' model of care, which the WHO describes as intrinsic to the provision of good medical care. In this model, psychological, spiritual, social, and physical concerns overlap, and problems in any one modality will impact on the others. Thus spiritual distress may increase physical breathlessness, and breathlessness may increase anxiety.

The multidisciplinary team needs to ensure that all dimensions are addressed for patients to receive the highest quality of care. Intractable 'total pain', for example, rarely responds fully to care in the physical domain only, such as analgesia. Focus on spiritual and psychological matters, such as the patient's interpretation of the meaning of the pain, can have a significant and positive impact on pain control.

Relieving distress

As people approach death, emotional defences tend to weaken. Personal issues that individuals may have previously been able to contain with the distractions of a busy life may become intrusive and troubling. Examples include previous unexplored grief, a past painful love affair, lost love, miscarriage, abortion, or sexual abuse. The dramatic emotional force that can be associated with such issues can cause profound distress, not least because the surfacing of the issue was so unexpected.

Making decisions

Religious or philosophical beliefs may have a direct impact on how a patient understands and responds to their illness and treatments. Important decisions may be affected, for example in relation to accepting or refusing life-prolonging interventions. This can cause particular tension when such beliefs run contrary to what the clinical team feel is appropriate.

Coping with adversity

There is increasing evidence that spiritual beliefs can be very supportive for patients and relatives going through the difficulties of life-threatening illness and imminent death.[1,2] Supporting patients to address spiritual concerns and to try to make sense of their situation can contribute to resilience and enhance coping.

Principles of care provision

Three dimensions of humanness

Every person is in certain respects:
- Like all others, human nature—universal
- Like some others, culture—local
- Like no other, personality—individual.

(Kluckhohn and Murray)[3]

A superficial response to cultural and spiritual need involves interpreting it as completion of a series of processes, achieved once a certain number of boxes have been ticked (e.g. priest called, imam informed). With such an approach, it is easy to lose sight of the individuality of the patient as a human who may have seemingly contradictory beliefs that cannot be dealt with by an easily defined system. It also overlooks the fact that the patient and the family may have different beliefs. Cultural and spiritual tensions can have an adverse impact on family cohesion and response to illness at this important time.

The intrinsic individuality of spiritual and cultural belief and practice should prevent inappropriate assumptions from being made. Some Jewish people eat pork. Some Catholics do not go to Mass. Some Muslims drink alcohol. Healthcare professionals should never stereotype spiritual identity, and individual assessment needs to be carried out.

Dying patients tend to be restricted to their place of care and often lack the physical strength to seek help from outside sources. Access to 'spiritual' expertise may therefore be limited. In practice, patients often seek spiritual or cultural affirmation from the professional staff looking after their physical needs. Regardless of the tradition or culture, patients can draw spiritual and cultural comfort from being treated with respect and care. Whilst it is seldom the responsibility of the clinical team to offer direct spiritual or cultural advice, it is always their responsibility to listen attentively to issues that are of concern to their dying patients. Where appropriate and with the patient's consent, referral may then be made to a suitable spiritual adviser.

References

1. Walsh K, King M, Jones L, Tookman A, Blizard R (2002) Spiritual beliefs may affect outcome of bereavement: prospective study. *Brit Med J*; 324 (7353): 1551.
2. Williams AL (2006) Perspectives on spirituality at the end of life: a meta-summary. *Palliat Support Care*; 4 (4): 407–417.
3. Murray MA, Kluckhohn C. Personality in Nature, Society and Culture. Revised 2nd edition 1953. Published by Knopf: New York.

Assessing spiritual needs

Communication skills

The clinician needs to establish a warm, confiding, professional rapport and convey clearly that the patient's priorities are at the centre of the agenda. As when taking a history about other potentially sensitive areas, if the clinician is not embarrassed about discussing the matter, then patients will tend not to be either.

However, some patients and staff, particularly those from reserved cultures, may find being asked and asking questions about spiritual beliefs intrusive. As always, communication will be influenced by the context and must be undertaken with sensitivity and respect for autonomy.

The key skill in conducting a spiritual and cultural 'needs assessment' is active listening. Careful listening to the patient's story will often provide the opportunity to ask questions. Such questions should be open in nature, giving the patient the chance to move the conversation in a direction of their choice.

Communication triggers

Reflecting on adversity

Patients' narratives invariably touch on their burdens and suffering. This can provide an opportunity to consider spiritual matters: 'You have been through so much recently…'

- '…what keeps you going?' or
- '…how have you kept going through all this?' or
- '…what has kept you going through all this?'

The patient may then express, for example, that they feel that it is their religious belief that has sustained them, or their love for their family, or a particular philosophical outlook. This can provide the clinician with an opportunity to assess gently the nature of these support systems and to consider how the team could provide additional support for the patient.

Existential questions

Many patients and carers confronting life-threatening or chronic intractable illness ask themselves the following types of questions:

- Why me?
- Why did it happen to me now?
- Am I punished for something?
- I feel guilty or responsible for what is happening to me (often important in people who smoke).
- Does my life mean anything?
- Have I achieved anything of worth in my life?
- Is it worth going on living like this?
- What will happen to my family?
- How will I die?
- Is there an existence after death?

These questions tend to be outward manifestations of inner spiritual turmoil. In a busy clinical context, it is easy to let such comments pass. In practice, however, these important questions tend to provide an ideal opportunity to explore spiritual concerns.

Advance care planning

Care planning discussions can provide another opportunity to assess spiritual needs:

- 'Is there anything particular that is worrying you?'
- 'What do you feel is happening?'
- 'What do you think is happening?'

Intractable symptoms

A full assessment of complex pain or other 'difficult symptoms' should always include questions to uncover spiritual and cultural distress.

> A 64-year-old lady with lung cancer was complaining of low central chest pain. The features of the pain were typical of gastritis, and she was commenced on omeprazole. Her pain, however, continued unabated and she was becoming increasingly distressed by it.
>
> A clinician eventually asked her what she thought was the cause of the pain. She whispered that she knew that it was believed to be coming from her stomach, but she was convinced that the pain meant that the cancer had come back and she was going to die. This led to a long conversation explaining the reasons why the pain was unlikely to be malignant in origin, and acknowledging and addressing her fears about the future. Her chest pain resolved completely that day.

Religious symbols

The patient's own use of religious symbols, such as the fish, the rosary, holy pictures, and sacred texts such as the Bible or Koran, may provide a trigger for sensitive questioning:

- 'Is your faith important to you?'

Spiritual assessment tool

Although a series of rote questions can never fully assess spiritual or cultural needs, it can be very helpful to have a few questions in mind that can enable the subject to be opened up in a non-intrusive manner.

Two examples of spiritual assessment tools are given in Tables 13.2 and 13.3. The ideas for ways of phrasing potentially sensitive questions can be useful, even when the tools are not themselves being used.

Avoiding assumptions

While it is worth taking note of any record of expressed spiritual belief or religious practice, it is important not to make assumptions about what that means to the patient. Recording 'Roman Catholic' on the nursing notes may mean, for example, that the patient wants a Christian burial or likes to use a rosary, but does not necessarily imply that they want to see a priest or receive the Last Rites.

When a patient describes him/herself as belonging to a particular religious group, it *cannot* be assumed that they:

- will be an orthodox practitioner of that religion
- want their support from a minister of that religion
- believe in the tenets of that religion; attachment may be cultural rather than religious.

Table 13.2 FICA: A Spiritual Assessment Tool[1]

F: Faith and Belief	Do you consider yourself spiritual or religious (if not, what gives you meaning?)
I: Importance	What importance does your faith or belief have in your life?
C: Community	Are you part of a spiritual or religious community?
A: Address/Action in care	What needs to be done with this information?

Table 13.3 The HOPE questions[2]

H: Sources of hope, meaning, comfort, strength, love and connection	• What do you hold onto during difficult times? • What sustains you and keeps you going? • For some people, their religious and spiritual beliefs act as a source of comfort and strength in dealing with life's ups and downs; is this true for you?
O: Organised religion	• Do you consider yourself part of an organised religion? • What aspects of your religion are helpful and not so helpful for you? • Are you part of a religious or spiritual community? Does it help you? How?
P: Personal spirituality and practices	• Do you have personal spiritual beliefs that are independent of organized religion? What are they? • What aspects of your spirituality or spiritual practices do you find most helpful to you personally? (eg prayer, reading scripture, listening to music)
E: Effects on medical care and end of life issues	• Has being sick affected your ability to do the things that usually help you spiritually? • As a doctor, is there anything that I can do to help you access the resources that usually help you? • Are you worried about any conflicts between your beliefs and your medical situation/care/decisions?

References

1. Post SG, Puchalski CM, Larson DB (2000) Physicians and patient spirituality: professional boundaries, competency, and ethics. *Ann Intern Med*; 132: 578–583.
2. Anandarajah G, High E (2001) Spirituality and medical practice: using the HOPE questions as a practical tool for spiritual assessment. *Am Fam Phys*; 63: 81–88.

Practical provision of care

Multidisciplinary team support

If a clinician identifies an important spiritual or cultural concern, it does not mean that he or she necessarily has to 'fix it.' Many such concerns cannot be easily solved, but need to be held and acknowledged. Other members of the multidisciplinary team, such as a chaplain, are usually best able to support patients with such issues.

- Hospital chaplains will try to involve ministers or clergymen of other denominations or religions if appropriate.
- A significant amount of their work is with patients with no firm belief system or atheists.
- Even when religion is not of importance to a patient, it may be that their carer or other family members require spiritual support.
- As always, patient confidentiality is vital and sensitive issues should not usually be shared within the team without patient consent.

Understanding customs

It is helpful for clinicians to have some understanding of the main customs and rituals of specific faiths (see Table 13.4 and 'Further reading'). For example, knowledge about specific religious holidays can help a patient celebrate in the hospital or go home to spend time with family. Nursing teams should be aware of important rituals after death. Some religions, such as Orthodox Judaism, do not support routine post mortem examinations (unless legally required), and great sensitivity is required should it become necessary to discuss such matters.

Avoid displaying knowledge of rituals as a route into discussion about spiritual needs. Individuals may not observe Passover or Ramadan or Lent in the manner in which the clinician understands them. Patients may then feel irrational guilt or perceive an implicit suggestion of shortcomings in their religious or spiritual practice. If, for example, a dying person of Muslim faith is asked about the Haj and has not been able to go (and now never will), this may contribute to distress.

Respecting individuality

'I am who I am and that is all right.'

Cicely Saunders

People approaching the end of life seem to want to achieve a sense of acceptance about themselves and their lives. This is a very personal journey, usually taken apart from even their family and closest friends.

At times, individuals choose to behave in a way that, although it may not seem to be in their best interest, remains important to them. For example, a patient may want to die at home, in what may appear to be relative squalor, when they could be in a clean hospital or hospice bed.

Although people usually wish for reconciliation with estranged family, on occasion people may make a choice to remain apart and angry. It is reasonable to offer patients who are clearly unhappy and angry spiritual support on a number of occasions. However, at some point it may become necessary to accept the individual's choice not to be reconciled. Such acceptance can in itself bring some comfort to a patient.

Health carers and family tend to find it very disturbing when a patient refuses to accept help. Support may then need to be mostly directed to the team and to the family, who may be harbouring long-standing regrets or distress about their relative's attitude or beliefs.

It is not possible to create meaning for another individual. The clinician's role is to help patients and carers receive the support that may allow them to find meaning themselves.

Supporting the healthcare team

Health carers may, at times, experience spiritual distress when caring for some patients. Particular issues arising during that care may resonate profoundly with personal experience. A perceptive and wise senior clinician can usually deal with such matters quietly and effectively.

When care for an individual patient has raised significant spiritual and cultural issues, it is helpful for the team to have the opportunity to reflect on the situation, in order to learn from the experience and also obtain a degree of closure. With the ever-growing cultural and spiritual diversity of modern life there will be much to learn in forthcoming years.

A number of attributes are prerequisites for clinicians to provide good cultural and spiritual care:

- Ability to accept others having religious beliefs, even if this appears to them to be in conflict with the scientific basis of medicine.
- Willingness to understand and work with people that are guided by a secular philosophy, when they are theist.
- Ability to work with and respect different cultural traditions.
- Willingness to accept that cultural and religious factors may have an impact on patient well-being and medical outcomes.
- When uncertain how to approach or manage spiritual concerns, willingness to seek help from someone who can.

Clinicians who do not have these attributes will require support, which may include cultural and religious diversity training.

Key points

- Spirituality is an important part of the human condition and it cannot be overlooked in clinical care.
- Dying people are often preoccupied by the need to find meaning in their lives.
- Physical and psychological distress can relate to spiritual and cultural concerns.
- Clinicians need to feel confident about asking about spirituality in its broadest sense.
- Key skills include the ability to create a warm, confiding rapport, use open questions, and listen actively.
- Clinicians need to know where to find spiritual, religious, or philosophical support for their patients.

Table 13.4 Common death rituals (Reproduced with permission)[1]

Hinduism	• Cremation occurs on a pyre by the river or at a crematorium by the evening of the day of death, and the ashes scattered. • Prayers and rituals occur on certain days within the first month. • Mourning period is 10 to 30 days.
Chinese traditions	• Elaborate funeral rituals occur at wakes lasting an odd number of days. • Chanting is undertaken by Buddhist or Taoist monks; paper effigies of money, clothes, houses, cars and other items needed in the afterlife are burned. • Wealthy are buried in a grand coffin after a funeral procession. • Observances or rituals occur at 7, 21, 49, and 100 days. • Mourning may last until the end of funeral or for 100 days, 1 year or 3 years, depending on the individual or family.
Buddhists	• Some do not wish the body to be disturbed for 8 hours or longer after death. • Buddhists have simpler funerals than Taoists (e.g. no burning of paper effigies). • Chanting is provided by Buddhist monks, if affordable by the family. • Cremation is favoured, but burial is acceptable. • Ashes may be stored at a columbarium in a temple.
Muslims	• Ritual washing is performed by family members of the same gender. • Burial occurs in a shroud within the body facing Mecca on the day of death before sundown.
Christians	• Simple rites are adapted to the local custom (e.g., a wake if it is the local practice). • Memorial services occur on the nights of the wake, at the funeral, burial or cremation, and sometimes at a later date. • Some Christians advocate burial; otherwise, cremation is done according to local practices. Roman Catholics have funeral masses and prefer burial.
Judaism	• Body should not be left alone from time of death until burial that takes place as soon as possible. • Body of the deceased is washed and dressed for burial, following specific ritual. • Traditionally, psalms are read beside body, a duty which can be performed by family members, friends or members of synagogue. • The burial is conducted with the reading of the "mourners' prayer". • Mourning takes place in several periods, each successively less intense, over a period of about 30 days. • Mourning begins with a 7-day period during which mourners are visited at home by family and community.

Reference

1. Goh CR (2008) Culture, ethnicity and illness. In Walsh TD, Caraceni AT, Fainsinger R et al (eds) *Palliative Medicine* pp. 51–55. Philadelphia, PA: Saunders/Elsevier.

Further reading

Database of patient experiences in the UK: www.healthtalkonline.org

NHS education for Scotland (2007) *A Multi-faith Resource for Healthcare Staff.* http://www.nes.scot.nhs.uk/media/7219/march07finalversions.pdf.pdf

Puchalski C (2009) Spiritual care. In: Walsh TD, Caraceni AT, Fainsinger R, *et al.* (eds.), *Palliative Medicine*. Elsevier Saunders, Philadelphia.

Strang S, Strang P (2009) Spiritual care. In: Bruera E, Higginson IJ, Ripamonti C, von Gunten C (eds.), *Textbook of Palliative Medicine*. Hodder Arnold, London.

The WHOQOL Group (1995) The WHO Quality of Life Assessment Position Paper from the World Health Organization. *Soc Sci Med*; 41: 1403–1409.

Caring for the carers

Introduction

'Too often carers are left to their own devices and do not come forward and admit they need support. Health workers don't always think to ask if there is any help or support they need.'
Views of a carer responding to NCPC survey, 2007[1]

This chapter considers the importance of caring for carers, both family and healthcare professionals. Although most of the chapter considers family carers, it is important to reflect on the demands on professionals, not least to ensure that patients get the best care.

Common characteristics of the carers of people with advanced respiratory disease are outlined in Table 14.1. There is increasing evidence that carers suffer from a multitude of physical and psychological problems, which are often hidden, both from the person they are caring for and from clinical services. There is even evidence for increased mortality in carers. Despite this, caring for carers is often not seen as an area in which clinicians should be interested, and health commissioners tend not to fund initiatives to help carers.

Healthcare professionals do not usually have a defined role or responsibilities for the patient's carers. In addition, carers may not be registered with the same GP practice as the patient, and clinicians have no authority to make a referral on their behalf. However, it is still important to consider the needs of the carer for a number of reasons:

- It is clear that caring for someone with advanced disease can have a damaging impact on carers' health, which may not be appreciated by others.
- The effectiveness of the care regimen for patients living at home is greatly influenced by their carer. Supporting the carer helps the patient.
- Healthcare professionals aim to reduce suffering and therefore should be concerned for the carer. This is central to the tenets of palliative care.

Emotional consequences of caring

Being a carer is a difficult role. Carers often experience a range of emotions as outlined below.

Frustration

It is frustrating being unable to undertake your usual enjoyable activities because of the constraints imposed by the patient's illness. Carers may also become frustrated with not knowing how to manage the patient, the patient's condition, or their own mental and physical well-being.

Anger

It is not unusual for carers to feel angry with the person they are caring for, who in turn may reciprocate because of their own distress. Carers may be angered if the person fails to comply with medical or other clinical advice. Anger frequently arises from the frustration of both parties with the new restrictions imposed on their lives and the loss of previous independence through different interests and work.

Exhaustion

Carers often feel exhausted because of carrying out not only their own tasks of everyday living but also all that used to be done by their relative. In addition, their spouse/relative may require physical care. These circumstances may last for years, requiring carers to find ways to pace themselves.

Anxiety

Carers may have an illness of their own and may worry that they are neglecting their own health. They may have other family members or friends with physical or psychological problems and wish to attend to them. Carers often feel isolated and overburdened, with no prospect of physical or psychological relief.

Distress

Carers may be distressed by the physical and psychological state of their relative. It can cause anguish watching a person one loves experiencing breathlessness, fatigue, or pain. They may feel distressed by their perception of their own helplessness. Others may feel distressed by their own feelings of exasperation and frustration with the situation.

Guilt

Feelings of guilt occur commonly. Carers may feel that they do not do enough, and that they cannot be the ideal 'loving and caring' carer that they imagine other people are in the same situation. They may feel guilty that at times they wish they could escape from the situation, or even that they may be feeling that life would be easier if their partner/relative was dead.

Fear

It is normal to feel frightened when caring for a person who is very breathless or in pain, particularly if the carer feels unable to do anything to improve the situation. Carers may fear that the person is about to stop breathing and wonder what to do should this happen. They may begin to dread weekends and bank holidays, when they perceive there is less medical support. They can feel isolated and fearful at the thought of having to cope with an emergency alone.

Bitterness

Carers may occasionally feel bitter about what has happened to them in life, about what they may see as the self-inflicted nature of their relative's illness, and about the lack of help they perceive they are getting from the NHS, friends, or society in general.

Depression

It is not uncommon for carers to become clinically depressed. They may experience feelings of worthlessness and guilty ruminations and may no longer be experiencing any pleasure in life.

Caring can, however, engender positive emotions too.

Pride

Carers may feel proud of what they are doing and the fact that no one else can do the job as well as they can. They may feel 'special' because of their extensive knowledge and understanding of their relative, and may feel pride at how they are managing a difficult situation.

Self-efficacy

Carers may develop feelings of self-belief and competence from caring. They may have mastered the intricacies of the health system and become skilled in talking to members of the medical, nursing, paramedical, and social services. They may feel a great sense of achievement from what they have learned by looking after their relative.

Table 14.1 Characteristics of carers

Characteristic	Comments
Majority are female	Many will already have caring role for children and/or elderly parents
Usually over 60 years	May find the physical burden of caring overwhelming, and can have own their health problems
Many not working	Inability to work because of caring role can lead to lower income and inability to afford extra help or support
Lacking information	Usually will not have attended pulmonary rehabilitation, and will have received less education about the disease than the patient
Constrained social life	Social isolation and loneliness are common consequences, particularly when caring over many years
Psychological morbidity	Distress, fear, anger and exhaustion can contribute to the development of anxiety and depression
Own needs suppressed	Reluctance to express own needs, because of prioritising those of the patient, can lead to resentment
Needs not known	May not be registered with the same practice as the patient, so the GP may be unaware of the carer's burden and strain

Reference

1. The National Council for Palliative Care (2009) *A Fresh Approach: Palliative and end of life care for people with Chronic Respiratory Disease*. www.ncpc.org.uk/policy_unit/circ_resp_pg.html.

Support for carers

'Our vision is that carers will be respected as expert care partners and will have access to the integrated and personalized services they need to support them in their caring role.'

Department of Health, 2008

Although some research has addressed specific interventions targeted towards carers, few definitive conclusions can be drawn. The following points, however, may help health professionals support their patients' carers.

Personalized support

Carers should be treated as individuals with individual needs and not simply as an extension of the caring team. It is easy but misguided to view their role as developing knowledge about the illness and carrying out allotted tasks, in order to spare the clinical team and keep the person out of hospital. A proportion of carers may not wish to be involved in clinical matters and this should be respected.

The support needs of a carer and the person being cared for may be quite different. For example, a patient may not like to talk about their illness and the future, whereas their carer may wish to discuss such matters frequently in order to express their grief and fears. Under such circumstances, organizing specific professional support for the carer with their permission, such as from a community nurse specialist or general practitioner, can be highly effective.

It is important not to view the patient and carer as an isolated unit. Many carers are concurrently supporting other family members such as elderly parents, children, and vulnerable adults. If this is occurring, it is important to explore alternative routes of support, so that one individual does not have to carry multiple burdens single-handed.

Practical support

Carers need to be able, as far as is possible, to have a life of their own outside of their caring role. It is important to find ways of creating time for carers to undertake activities that are of importance to them.

Respite care is a scarce resource in most parts of the UK. On occasion, patients with advanced disease may be admitted to a hospice for symptom control, but the underlying reason is primarily to support an exhausted carer.

Extra support from paid or voluntary carers in the home can be arranged. The patient's daily routine does not have to be significantly disrupted, a potential source of great anxiety, and the carer can be liberated to leave the home for a day or even take a holiday.

Overall, the most important part of caring for carers is recognizing that they are individuals with needs of their own. Although primary attention is focused on the needs of the patient, spending time talking with the carer in private, acknowledging the challenges of their role and suggesting options for support, can effectively help both the patient and their carer.

Carers of patients attending the Breathlessness Intervention Service in Cambridge, UK, use the patients' 'well-being mindfulness intervention' as much as the patients themselves do.

Table 14.2 Sources of support

Source	Comments
High quality patient care	Optimisation of the patient's health significantly helps the carer as well as the patient. Creating effective out of hours support is of particular value.
Unbureaucratic clinical support	Repeat prescriptions delivered to the home, organised transport to appointments, and home visits can greatly reduce the demands on the carer.
Self-help groups	Breathe Easy support groups (British Lung Foundation), cancer support groups and other disease specific groups can be very helpful, providing social support as well as information.
Befriending services	Befriending throughout the illness trajectory, often by volunteers, appears to lead to a reduced need for subsequent bereavement support.
Family and psychological support services	Burdens placed on carers can put strain on marital and family relationships, leading to unhappiness and tension at home.
Primary health care team	The carers' health must be attended to, particularly, as is common in elderly carers, if they have their own medical condition.
Home carers	Carers can come from statutory social services, private sources and charities, such as Crossroads Care. It is helpful to encourage carers to use the time for recreation, rather than practical tasks.
Respite care	Some residential or nursing homes provide respite care, but it is rarely free. Hospice and other day centres can also give carers valuable hours of respite.
Financial support	This is often needed, particularly when carers have had to leave paid employment. Carers may be entitled to a range of social security benefits, as well as flexible employment opportunities.

Bereavement support

Grief is a journey to a new normality.

Healthcare professionals must be familiar with and confident in responding to the grief of families and friends and facilitating appropriate support. Grief is a normal process that occurs after a major loss, with a broad range of manifestations including physical, cognitive, and behavioural, as well as emotional, consequences.

Models of grief

The theoretical models of the grieving process have value in giving those supporting grieving people a conceptual understanding of what they are witnessing. Worden[1] describes grief as a process during which a number of tasks need to be accomplished:

- To accept the reality of loss.
- To experience and work through the pain of grief.
- To adjust to an environment where the deceased is no longer present.
- To emotionally relocate the deceased and move on with life.

Another useful model is the Dual Process Model of Stroebe and Schut[2]. This recognizes that grief is a dynamic process where bereaved people oscillate between focusing on the loss of the person ('loss orientation') and avoiding that focus ('restoration orientation'). Both states are necessary for future adjustment, although people tend to become more restoration focused with time.

Klass et al.[3] suggest that the purpose of grieving, rather than 'breaking bonds' with the deceased and moving on, is to maintain a continuing bond that is compatible with new and ongoing relationships.

Bereavement care

Less than half of the carers of patients with chronic non-malignant respiratory disease have access to bereavement support.

NCPC survey, 2008[4]

The essence of bereavement support is to help individuals tell their story. According to the models above, grief is a process or journey, which can be helped by facilitating people to engage with their loss and work through it. People are helped by:

- being able to express their feelings, with affirmation of their reality and legitimacy
- sharing memories of past experiences with that person, reflecting on their attributes, qualities, and quirks
- reassurance that they need not and will not forget the deceased but can integrate that person into their future lives with a continuing bond
- finding ways to make sense of the past and guidance towards a meaningful future.

Although giving time and listening to bereaved individuals is of the greatest value, a degree of support can be given by the information contained in bereavement leaflets. These can outline and validate the normal feelings associated with grief and describe the journey through grief ahead. Leaflets can also include details of sources of future support such as:

- local counselling and psychological support services
- bereavement services run by specialist palliative care teams
- the National Bereavement Service in the UK
- charities such as Cruse and Compassionate Friends.

Complicated grief

Mourning is a normal and essential adaptive response to loss. Complicated grief is said to occur where there is a continuation of grief-related manifestations beyond a time that is considered adaptive. It can lead to enduring psychological, social, and physical morbidity.

Risk factors

Risk factors for complicated grief include the following:

- sudden or unexpected death
- multiple past losses
- anxious personality and/or low self-esteem
- overly dependent or, conversely, ambivalent relationship with the deceased
- family dysfunction, isolation, or alienation
- child, teenager, or young dependent adult at time of loss
- male over 55 years who will be living alone after the loss. This group is at higher risk of suicide in the first 2 years after bereavement.

Healthcare professionals should make particular efforts to ensure that those at risk of complicated grief get follow-up support, with encouragement to make links with formal support services. It is important to gain permission to contact their GP if they are at a different practice from the patient. The GP may have no knowledge of the difficulties that the patient and carers have been through.

Reducing risk

Clinicians can reduce the risk of complicated grief in a number of ways.

- Keep relatives and carers up to date with the patient's condition and anticipate questions. Many people are still hesitant to ask about important changes in a patient's physical state. A point that is obvious to a medically trained person (such as that a person is dying) may come as a shock to carers.
- Ensure that the patient has good symptom control. Watching a person die with intractable breathlessness or pain can leave the observer with significant psychological problems, including post-traumatic stress disorder (PTSD).
- Predict who may be at high risk and refer early for specialist help. Explaining why an individual is at risk may facilitate acceptance of help.

References

1. Worden JW. Grief counselling and grief therapy: A handbook for the mental health practitioner, 2nd ed. New York, NY: Springer Publishing co; 1991.
2. Shoebe M, Schut H. The dual process model of coping with bereavement: rationale and description. Death Studies 1999; 23: 197–224.
3. Klass D, Silverman S, Nickman S (eds) Continuing bonds: new understandings of grief. Washington: Taylor and Francis; 1996.
4. The National Council for Palliative Care (2009) A Fresh Approach: Palliative and end of life care for people with Chronic Respiratory Disease. www.ncpc.org.uk/policy_unit/circ_resp_pg.html

Caring for professionals

Clinicians caring for people with advanced disease must learn how to continue to care and be empathetic, without absorbing too much of the distress and anguish encountered during clinical work. Although, of course, it is vital to avoid becoming a seemingly heartless clinician interested only in the pathophysiology of disease, it is equally damaging to patients and carers to be an 'over-involved' clinician, needy for praise, who eventually succumbs to physical or mental ill-health.

Factors associated with burnout

There are many factors that appear to increase the risk of emotional exhaustion.

- Unremitting contact with human suffering and distress.
- Heavy workload, staff shortages, long hours, and erosion of home time.
- Complexity of clinical workload, regularly facing emergency situations.
- Heavy emotional load and demanding patients and family members.
- Poor team management or organization and lack of institutional support.
- Poor relationships with colleagues; tension within the healthcare team.
- Lack of recognition of effort from colleagues and team leaders.
- Lack of control over working conditions, with restrictions and inadequate resources hindering ability to perform one's role well.
- Relative lack of competence or experience in the role.
- Use of cigarettes, alcohol, or medication as a means of relaxation.
- Poor work-life balance, with limited time for home life and interests.
- Challenges in own social life and lack of support from family or friends.

Staying healthy

This relies on having a personal commitment and drive towards remaining healthy. A number of factors can help.

- Ensure that patients with challenging problems are shared within the healthcare team. Avoid taking sole responsibility for every aspect of a patient's care.
- Try to develop control over daily work, including flexible working patterns.
- Optimize professional effectiveness, so reducing the need to work prolonged hours.
- Encourage any activities that can improve team support and lead to team building. Peer support can have a highly significant impact on relieving distress.
- Avoid physical exhaustion and prioritize getting sufficient sleep.
- Maintain an interesting and diverse life outside work.
- Maintain physical fitness, with a healthy diet and exercise regimen, and avoid using alcohol, cigarettes, or medication to aid relaxation.
- Attend to personal health needs and be registered with a GP.
- Become self-aware, developing insight into when one is living unhealthily or becoming psychologically distressed.
- Actively seek support when under strain, including professional support when needed.

- Establish which forms of support are personally most helpful, such as team meetings, regular contact with a colleague in another centre, or formal support from a psychologist.

Further reading

Booth S, Edmonds P, Kendall M (2009) Personal survival. In: Booth S, Edmonds P, Kendall M, *Palliative Care in the Acute Hospital Setting: A practical guide*. Oxford University Press, Oxford.

Butler G, Hope T (1995) *Manage Your Mind: The mental fitness guide*. Oxford University Press, Oxford.

Booth S, Burkeu J, Moffat C (2010). Cambridge Breathlessness Intervention Service Manual. Cambridge University Hospitals NHS Foundation Trust http://www.cuh.org.uk/breathlessness.

Currow D, Ward A, Clark K, Burns C, Abernathy A (2008) Caregivers for people with end-stage lung disease: characteristics and unmet needs in the whole population. *International Journal of COPD*; 3 (4): 753–762.

Department of Health (2008) *Carers at the Heart of 21st-century Families and Communities. A caring system at your side. A life of your own*. DH Publications, London.

Simpson A, Young J, Donahue M, Rocker G (2010) A day at a time: caregiving on the edge in COPD. *International Journal of COPD*; 5: 141–151.

Index